ISBN: 9798655365285

30-DAY
Mediterranean
Diet

Vincent Antonetti, PhD
Tina Hudson, MS

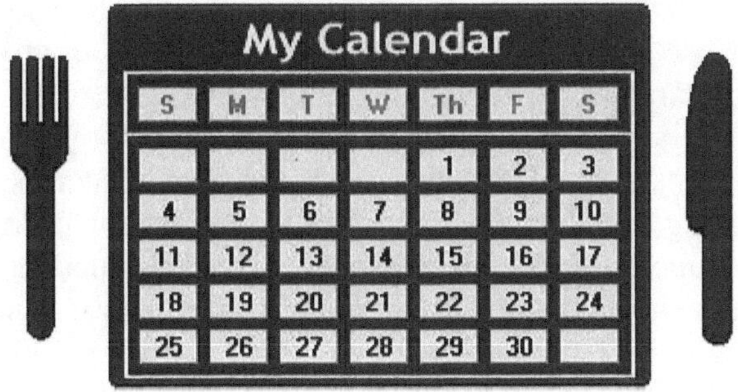

NoPaperPress™

Note: At publication, the off-the-shelf foods used in some of this book were widely available in most supermarkets. But food products come and go. So if there is a frozen entrée or soup selection in this diet that is out of stock, or that's been discontinued, or perhaps you don't like, or that you forgot to pick up while shopping, please substitute another food that has **approximately** the same caloric value.

PREFACE

In 1958, Ancel Keys, a highly-regarded scientist at the University of Minnesota, started a landmark research project of healthy middle-aged men called The Seven Countries Study[1]. The project lasted decades and included men living in Greece, Italy, Yugoslavia, the Netherlands, Finland, and the United States. His findings supported previous studies that pointed to saturated fats as the cause of the arterial blockages that resulted in heart disease and heart attacks. But he also found that in Mediterranean countries, such as Greece and Italy, heart disease was not as prevalent and caused fewer deaths than in northern Europe and the United States. Dr. Keys was the first to advocate the health implications of a Mediterranean-style diet.

Generally speaking the Mediterranean diet is a way of eating based on the long-established cuisine of the countries bordering the Mediterranean Sea. The diet typically contains lots of vegetables, fruits, whole grain breads, beans, seafood, nut and seeds, olive oil and red wine. Plant-based foods are central to the diet. But moderate amounts of dairy, seafood, poultry and eggs are also important in the Mediterranean Diet. In contrast, red meat is eaten infrequently.

Healthy fats are a mainstay of a Mediterranean diet and are consumed instead of unhealthy saturated and trans fats which contribute to heart disease. Olive oil is the primary source of added fat in a Mediterranean diet. Olive oil is a monounsaturated fat, which has been found to lower total cholesterol and LDL (or "bad") cholesterol levels. Nuts and seeds also contain monounsaturated fat.

Seafood is also important in the Mediterranean diet. Fatty fish such as mackerel, herring, sardines, albacore tuna, salmon and lake trout, all rich in omega-3 fatty acids, a type of polyunsaturated fat that is thought to reduce inflammation in humans. Omega-3 fatty acids also help to decrease triglycerides, reduce blood clotting, and decrease the risk of stroke and congestive heart failure. A typical Mediterranean diet allows red wine - but only in moderation.

Research has shown that the Mediterranean Diet is by far one of the healthiest in the world. It's important to note that the Mediterranean Diet in this book is also a **Reducing Diet** and therefore shows the caloric value of the foods in the diet. In fact, what makes the Mediterranean Diet in this book different is the emphasis on calorie control which is what leads directly to weight loss.

The version of the Mediterranean Diet in this book has been modified slightly to be consistent with American dietary patterns, food preferences and calorie control.

Note that Vince (the primary author) is three-quarters Italian and Tina's mother was of Italian decent. This is the diet we both grew up eating.

Vince Antonetti & Tina Hudson
July 2020

---

1. Keys, Ancel. "Coronary problems in seven countries." Circulation 41.1 (1970): 186-195.

CONTENTS

1200 CALORIE MEAL PLANS

1500 CALORIE MEAL PLANS

RECIPIES & DIET TIPS

The Best Weight-Loss Diets

According to the late Dr. Jean Mayer of Harvard University's Department of Nutrition, a really good weight-loss diet must have the following three characteristics:

1) The diet must provide you with an understanding of weight control as well as the knowledge you need to reduce your weight to the desired level.
2) The diet must help you remain healthy while you are losing weight.
3) The diet must lead you to a healthier way of eating and exercising that will, in the long term, help you keep off the weight you have lost.

The Mediterranean weight-loss diet featured in this book is a diet that is not only low calorie and reasonably low in fat, but is also nutritionally balanced. The *30-Day Mediterranean Diet*, however, does not meet all the criteria set forth above. While you will acquire some "dieting insight" and some idea of how much you can eat and still lose weight, you will not get a real understanding of weight control from this book. That's not its purpose. What you will get is a healthy diet – and a diet that if followed will promote weight loss. Think of the *30-Day Mediterranean Diet* as a quick fix, a healthy start that will get you on the right track – but it's not the long-term answer.

Long-term success is about developing both an understanding and a plan that will result in healthier eating and physical activity habits. For a through understanding and the guidance you need to succeed in the long term we recommend you read, *Weight Control - U.S. Edition* by Vincent Antonetti, Ph.D., another NoPaperPress book.

Begin with a Medical Exam

Everyone should at the very least have a medical assessment, or exam, before starting a weight loss diet. Why? You need to make sure your health will allow you to lower your caloric intake and increase your physical activity. The medical checkup may be as simple as a visit to a physician who is familiar with your medical history, or it may be a thorough physical exam. The physician conducting the medical exam should be made aware of and should approve the specific weight loss diet you're planning.

What's in This Book?

This book actually contains two 30-day diets: an 1500 Calorie diet, and for even faster weight loss a 1200 Calorie diet. And both diets have a meal plan (menu) for each and every one of the 30 days.

Which Calorie Level is for You?

1200 Calorie Mediterranean Diet: Most women and smaller men, older men and inactive men should select this calorie level.

1500 Calorie Mediterranean Diet: This calorie level is for most men and larger women, younger women and active women.

How Much Weight Will You Lose?

Weight loss occurs when your food energy intake is less than the total energy you expend. This difference in calories is referred to as your <u>calorie deficit</u>. How much weight you lose depends on the magnitude of your calorie deficit. Simple metabolic calculations make a rough estimate possible.

On the 30-Day Mediterranean Diet, <u>most women lose 8 to 16 pounds</u> – depending on whether the 1500 or 1200 Calorie diet is selected.

On the 30-Day Mediterranean Diet, <u>most men lose 14 to 24 pounds</u> – depending on whether the 1500 or 1200 Calorie diet is selected.

Smaller adults, older adults and less active adults will lose a bit less and larger adults, younger adults and more active adults often much more. Exactly how much weight you will lose depends on how much you weigh, your age and your activity level. Again, for the full story see *Weight Control - U.S. Edition* by Vincent Antonetti, Ph.D.

Guidelines for Healthy Eating

Even though most adults can get all the vitamins and minerals they need by merely consuming a variety of nutritious foods (from the fruit group, the vegetable group, the grains group, the meat and beans group, the milk group, and the oils group), many physicians recommend a daily multi-vitamin/mineral supplement – just in case you don't eat the way you should.

<u>Large Salad:</u> One of the dinner mainstays is a "Large Salad." Prepare your "Large Salad" in a bowl with a volume of at least 16 ounces, or 2 cups. First add about 1 cup of either green leaf lettuce, Romaine lettuce or a mesclun mix. Then add, as desired, another cup of other veggies such as broccoli, celery, cucumber, tomato, onion, peppers, spinach, or watercress. This vegetable combination will, on average, total about 40 Calories. You will be eating a "Large Salad" just about every day at dinnertime. Remember that variety is the key to a nutritious diet. So be sure to vary the ingredients of the salad. Top your salad with <u>two tablespoons</u> of the following the salad dressing on the next page.

For a "**Small Salad**" use half the ingredients of the preceding large salad and half of the following salad dressing.

<u>Salad Dressing:</u> Mix two tablespoons of extra virgin olive oil (EVOO) with one tablespoon of balsamic vinegar and one tablespoon of water. Add salt, pepper and any Italian herbs to taste. Whisk ingredients together. Shake well. Use half of the dressing on your salad. Save the remainder in your fridge in a sealed container.

Your "Large Salad" with salad dressing will cost you roughly 150 Calories but will be packed with lots of health-giving vitamins, minerals and fiber.

<u>Homemade Cooking Spray:</u> Simply combine one part olive oil with one part water into a spray bottle. Shake well and spray! Cheap, low calorie and effective.

<u>Soup</u>: See page 114 for a list of the soup permitted on this diet. To improve the taste of canned soup, add a teaspoon of grated cheese before heating in a microwave oven. After heating, add ½ teaspoon of olive oil. Stir and serve. These additions total about 30 Calories but really enhance the taste.

<u>About Bread:</u> First understand that bread, more specifically whole-grain breads, are good sources of complex carbohydrates and dietary fiber, as well as several B vitamins (thiamin, riboflavin, niacin, and foliate), vitamin E, and minerals (iron, magnesium and selenium). In recent years, however, sliced bread loaves have gotten larger, as have the bread slices inside these loaves. Just a few years ago the standard slice of bread contained about 65 to 70 Calories – now most are 100 plus Calories.

The *30-Day Mediterranean Diet* requires whole-grain bread at 65 to 70 Calories per slice for breakfast toast. Quite a few bakers sell thin sliced or "light" sliced bread. The difficult part is finding a whole grain thin sliced or "light" bread (with about 70 Calories per slice). Whatever the brand, make sure the first word in the Ingredients list is "whole." "Pepperidge Farm Small Slice 100% Whole Wheat" is a good breakfast choice. It's whole grain, has 70 Calories per slice and it tastes good too.

For dinner find a good loaf of **Italian or French bread** and use about one ounce (80 Calories). <u>Hint</u>: Get the weight of the loaf from the label, or weigh it on a scale in the produce section of the store. Then estimate how many one ounce servings the loaf contains and slice accordingly.

Exchanging Foods

If there is a food listed in the *30-Day Mediterranean Diet* that you don't like, or perhaps that you forgot to pick up while shopping, you probably can exchange or substitute another food in its place – a technique used by dieticians. Exchanging a food listed in a diet for another food with approximately equal caloric value and nutritional content is the foundation of a successful long-term diet. Substitution possibilities are almost endless but have to be done carefully.

The easiest substitutions are those within the same food group, such as exchanging one vegetable variety for another, or a glass of milk for a cup of yogurt. More sophisticated exchanges cross food groups, for instance replacing 3½ ounces of turkey with a tablespoon of peanut butter spread on a piece of whole wheat bread. Both foods are complete protein and both contain about 175 Calories.

Refer to a good online calorie table. With some understanding and experience, you can use this table to help you substitute foods called for in the *30-Day Mediterranean Diet* with equal calorie foods from the same food group.

Breakfast: You may substitute any cereal for any other wholesome cereal. For example, if you're not crazy about having Shredded Wheat for breakfast on Day 6, substitute Wheat Chex or Cheerios, etc. If you don't like the soft-boiled egg called for on Day 9, make yourself a scrambled egg instead. And if Cantaloupe is on the menu but is not in season, replace the cantaloupe with a half cup of orange juice.

Snacks: Again, where yogurt is specified you may substitute a 6-ounce glass of skim milk, but to maintain a nutritionally balanced diet keep this snack a dairy selection. Similarly, when fruit is on the agenda, you may select another type of fruit but do not stray from the fruit group. Nuts and popcorn can be interchanged at will. (Incidentally, you should buy a hot-air popper. They make great popcorn – which is high in fiber and makes a tasty and nutritious snack.)

Two Nights Off

Everyone deserves a break from the grind of preparing dinner after coming home from work. So the *30-Day Mediterranean Diet* gives you two days off per week! Notice that one night a week the meal plan calls for a frozen dinner and on a second night during the week you're encouraged to eat out. There are, however, some rules and caveats involved and these are covered in the next two sections.

Frozen Dinners

In general, a frozen dinner should not be a meal in itself. Make sure you add a salad, fruit, bread etc. The frozen dinner you choose should come with at least one cup of cooked vegetables. If your frozen dinner doesn't measure up, add your own frozen, fresh or canned vegetables. And look for dinners with no more than 800 mg of sodium. In addition, make sure the dinner you choose has no more than 30 percent of the daily value for total fat. **Appendix A** lists almost 150 frozen dinner entrees.

And on the days when a frozen dinner is specified, you will also be given a calorie goal for the frozen dinner. For example, Day 5 calls for frozen fish dinner with a maximum allowable 300 Calories. If you choose a frozen fish dinner that contains less than 300 Calories, you may spend the unused calories any way you wish.

Moreover, on those nights when you just don't have the energy or time to cook, you can always substitute a frozen dinner for the entree listed in the meal plan. For example, Day 1 calls for Chicken with Peppers and Onions for dinner. The total calorie count for dinner is 500. In place of the chicken, any combination of a frozen chicken dinner and side dishes (salads, etc) with a total calorie content close to 500 would be an acceptable, albeit not as tasty, an alternative.

Eating Out

You may eat out once a week. When you're on a diet, however, eating in a restaurant can be a challenge, because most restaurant portions are huge, and can easily total more than 1,000 Calories. On the *30-Day Mediterranean Diet*, a dinner type (i.e., fish, chicken, etc) and a calorie target is specified. For example Day 7 of the 1500 Calorie diet specifies a chicken dinner and allows you 630 Calories.

First, you need to choose a restaurant where you have a fighting chance to achieve your calorie goal. Next, order simple, such as broiled chicken breast with steamed vegetables and brown rice. Tell the waiter you want no sauce, no gravy, nothing added. Then, knowing your calorie objective, and that most fish and chicken are about 50 Calories per ounce, most steamed vegetable servings average approximately 50 Calories per cup, and rice is about 100 Calories per ½ cup, decide how much to eat – and take the remainder home. If fresh fruit is not an option, pass on dessert and have the evening snack specified in the meal plan for that day.

Mediterranean Diet Info

As mentioned previously, there are two diet plans in this book:
 -.1200 Calorie 30-Day Diet starts on page 15.

- 1500 Calorie 30-Day Diet starts on page 46.
Both have a detailed meal plan for each of the 30 days. Associated with each day is a "Recipe of the Day" and a "Diet Tip of the Day."

After you complete the 30th day on the diet, if you still want to lose more weight a good option is to repeat the diet by starting over at Day 1.

Important Notes

1) Coffee may be decaf or regular. If desired, skim milk and a sugar substitute may be added to coffee or tea. And soy or almond milk may be used instead of cow's milk.

2) Fried eggs or scrambled eggs should be cooked in a pan coated with a non-stick cooking spray (see page 9). Hard-boiled eggs may be substituted for fried, scrambled or soft-boiled eggs.

3) Cereals should be whole grain and unsweetened. At the top of the list are Old-fashioned Oatmeal, Wheatena and Shredded Wheat. Among other reasonably healthy choices are Cheerios, Wheat Chex, Wheaties, some Kashi cereals and Farina. When blueberries are in season, you may add blueberries instead of raisins to your cereal. (Substitution ratio = 2 blueberries per raisin.)

4) Bread may be either plain or toasted whole grain, such as whole wheat, whole rye or pumpernickel. Look for whole grain varieties that contain 70 Calories per slice. If desired, bread may be topped with a home-made low-calorie olive oil spray. NO BUTTER!

5) When soup is specified, have only one serving (8 ounces) unless otherwise noted. (Most caned soups usually contain about two servings.)

6) Use freely as desired: clear unsweetened coffee, clear unsweetened tea, water, seltzer water and any diet soda, clear soups without fat, bouillon, and seasonings such as mustard, cinnamon, dill, herbs, red and black pepper, curry, vinegar, lemon juice and sections, and dill and sour pickles.

7) Use only lean cuts of meat trimmed of all visible fat. Poultry should be limited to chicken or turkey breasts (white meat only and skinless).

8) When canned tuna or salmon is specified, use only fish packed in water.

9) When the diet calls for turkey bacon, make sure the brand you buy has no more than 35 Calories per slice.

10) An unlimited amount of salad may be eaten, but the salad dressing should be as specified.

11) Use freely as desired: clear unsweetened coffee, clear unsweetened tea, water, seltzer, any diet soda, clear soups without fat, bouillon, and seasonings such as mustard, cinnamon, dill, herbs, red and black pepper, curry, vinegar, lemon juice and sections, and dill and sour pickles.

12) If it's more convenient, any food item may be moved to any part of the day and combined with any meal or snack.

13) If you cannot find the exact item called for in the diet (because it's out of stock or discontinued), substitute a comparable food (of the same type and close caloric value).

14) Although it's recommended that you follow the diet days as specified, it's fine to occasionally skip a day and/or pick and choose the days you prefer. (Nutritionally, each day stands on its own.)

1200-Calorie
Daily Menus

Day 1 – 1200 Calorie Meal Plan

BREAKFAST	Calories	Totals
Grapefruit (½)	75	
Scrambled egg (see Notes page 12)	80	
Whole-grain toast (1 slice) (see page 9)	65	
Coffee (Notes - page 12)	10	230 Cal
SNACK		
Coffee or tea	10	10 Cal
LUNCH		
Salad – 3 oz canned salmon, 1 tsp Evoo, onions & celery	200	
Lettuce & tomato wedges	20	
Italian or French bread (1 slice - see page 9)	80	
Water	0	300 Cal
SNACK		
Greek Yogurt (6 oz, nonfat, any flavor)*	90	90 Cal
DINNER		
Chicken w Peppers & Onions (Day 1 Recipe - page 77)	250	
Sautéed red peppers with onions	70	
Green beans (steamed) & mashed cauliflower	45	
Large salad with 2 Tbsp dressing (see page 9)	150	
Water	0	515 Cal
SNACK		
Fresh fruit in season (apple, plum, etc)	70	
* Such as, Dannon Lite & Fit. (Buy 32 oz container & use 6 oz.)		1215 Cal

Day 2 – 1200 Calorie Meal Plan

BREAKFAST	Calories	Totals
Fresh or frozen strawberries (½ cup)	25	
French toasted English Muffin (Day 2 Recipe - page 78)	270	
Light syrup (1 Tbsp)	30	
Coffee (Notes - page 12)	10	335 Cal
SNACK		
Coffee or tea	10	10 Cal
LUNCH		
Salad (3 oz tuna, 1 tsp Evoo, onions & celery)	175	
Lettuce & tomato wedges	20	
Italian or French bread (1 slice - see page 9)	80	
Hot or iced tea	10	285 Cal
SNACK		
Greek Yogurt (6 oz, nonfat, any flavor)	90	
Coffee or tea	10	100 Cal
DINNER		
Broiled veal chop (4 oz lean)	200	
Broccoli (½ cup steamed)	25	
Large salad with 2 Tbsp dressing (see page 9)	150	
Glass red wine (4 oz)	100	395 Cal
SNACK		
Fresh fruit in season (apple, peach, etc)	70	70 Cal
		1205 Cal

Day 3 – 1200 Calorie Meal Plan

BREAKFAST	Calories	Totals
Orange juice (½ cup)	50	
Wheaties (¾ cup) + ½ cup skim milk + ½ banana	190	
Coffee (See Notes page 12)	10	250 Cal
SNACK		
Fresh fruit in season (apple, peach, etc)	70	70 Cal
LUNCH		
Soup (Appendix C - page 114)*	110	
Turkey breast (1 oz) on 1 slice bread (½ sandwich)	105	
Lettuce & tomato slices	20	
Hot or ice tea	10	245 Cal
* 30 calories added to account for flavor enhancements.		
SNACK		
Coffee or tea	10	10 Cal
DINNER		
Baked Herb-Crusted Cod (Day 3 Recipe - page 79)	230	
Spinach (½ cup) steamed with garlic & drizzled Evoo	100	
Asparagus (7 spear cooked & drained)	20	
Italian or French bread (1 slice)	80	
Glass of red wine (4 oz)	100	
Water	0	530 Cal
SNACK		
Fiber One Chocolate Fudge Brownie	90	
Coffee or tea	10	100 Cal
		1205 Cal

Day 4 – 1200 Calorie Meal Plan

BREAKFAST	Calories	Totals
Grapefruit (½)	75	
Cheerios (1 cup) + ½ cup skim milk + about 15 raisins*	180	
Coffee	10	265 Cal
SNACK		
Coffee or tea	10	10 Cal
LUNCH		
Subway 6" (Roast Beef, Cheese + veggies)**	245	
Large salad with 2 Tbsp dressing	150	
Water	0	395 Cal
** On 6" half wheat roll.		
SNACK		
Fresh fruit in season (peach, plum, etc)	70	70 Cal
DINNER		
Pasta and Veggies (Day 4 Recipe - page 80)	460	
Water	0	460 Cal
SNACK		
Coffee or tea	10	10 Cal
* See page 10 re substituting blueberries for raisins.		1210 Cal

Day 5 – 1200 Calorie Meal Plan

BREAKFAST	Calories	Totals
Cantaloupe (½ medium)	50	
Fried egg	80	
Toasted raisin bread (1 slice)	75	
Coffee	10	215 Cal
SNACK		
Coffee or tea	10	10 Cal
LUNCH		
Soup (Appendix C - page 114)	140	
Italian or French bread (1 slice)	80	
Lettuce and sliced tomato with 1 Tbsp dressing	85	
Hot or iced tea	10	315 Cal
* 30 calories added to account for flavor enhancements.		
SNACK		
Greek Yogurt (6 oz, nonfat, any flavor)	90	90 Cal
DINNER		
Frozen fish dinner (Day 5 Recipe - page 81)	340	
Large salad with 2 Tbsp dressing	150	
Water	0	490 Cal
SNACK		
One small cookie*	80	
Coffee or tea	10	90 Cal
* Oatmeal, ginger snap, sugar, etc - check calories!		1210 Cal

Day 6 – 1200 Calorie Meal Plan

BREAKFAST	Calories	Totals
Tomato juice (½ cup)	20	
Shredded Wheat (1 cup) + ½ cup skim milk + ½ banana	265	
Coffee	10	295 Cal
SNACK		
Coffee or tea	10	10 Cal
LUNCH		
Ham (2 oz) with mustard on 2 slices rye bread	290	
Lettuce	10	
Hot or iced tea	10	310 Cal
SNACK		
Fresh fruit in season (pear, plum, etc)	70	70 Cal
DINNER		
Pizza (Day 6 Recipe - page 82)	350	
Large salad with 2 Tbsp dressing	150	
Hot or iced tea	10	500 Cal
SNACK		
Coffee or tea	10	10 Cal
		1195 Cal

Day 7 – 1200 Calorie Meal Plan

BREAKFAST	Calories	Totals
Cantaloupe (½ medium)	50	
Oatmeal (½ cup dry) + ½ cup skim milk + about 15 raisins	220	
Coffee	10	280 Cal
SNACK		
Coffee or tea	10	10 Cal
LUNCH		
Grilled cheese sandwich (2 slices 2% cheese)	230	
Lettuce and sliced tomato	20	
Water	0	250 Cal
SNACK		
Carrot sticks + ¼ cup low-fat cottage cheese & chives	60	60 Cal
DINNER		
Eat Out – Chicken dinner (Day 7 Recipe - page 83)	480	
Glass wine (4 oz)	100	580 Cal
SNACK		
Coffee or tea	10	10 Cal
		1190 Cal

Day 8 – 1200 Calorie Meal Plan

BREAKFAST	Calories	Totals
Cantaloupe (½ medium)	50	
Wheaties (¾ cup) + ½ cup skim milk + ½ banana	190	
Coffee	10	250 Cal
SNACK		
Coffee or tea	10	10 Cal
LUNCH		
Soup (Appendix C - page 114)*	120	
Turkey (1 oz) on 1 slice of rye bread (½ sandwich)	115	
Lettuce & tomato slices	20	
Hot or iced tea	10	265 Cal
* 30 calories added to account for flavor enhancements.		
SNACK		
Small bunch of grapes	65	65 Cal
DINNER		
Baked salmon with salsa (Day 8 Recipe - page 84)	215	
Summer squash, zucchini and tomatoes	60	
Brown rice (½ cup)	100	
Large salad with 2 Tbsp dressing	150	
Water with lemon wedge	10	535 Cal
SNACK		
Fresh fruit in season (apple, plum, etc)	70	70 Cal
		1195 Cal

Day 9 – 1200 Calorie Meal Plan

BREAKFAST	Calories	Totals
Orange juice (½ cup)	50	
Soft-boiled egg	80	
Whole-grain toast (1 slice)	65	
Coffee	10	205 Cal
SNACK		
Coffee or tea	10	10 Cal
LUNCH		
Salad (3 oz tuna, 1 tsp Evoo, onions & celery)	175	
Lettuce & tomato wedges	20	
Rye bread (1 slice)	65	
Fresh fruit in season (pear, peach, etc)	70	
Water or diet soda	0	330 Cal
SNACK		
Greek Yogurt (6 oz, nonfat, any flavor)	90	90 Cal
DINNER		
Veggie burger – (1 patty) (Day 9 Recipe - page 85)	100	
Low-fat cheddar cheese (1 thin slice)	50	
Seeded hamburger roll + Beets (3 small)	185	
Large salad with 2 Tbsp dressing	150	
Water	0	475 Cal
SNACK		
One small cookie	80	
Coffee or tea	10	90 Cal
		1200 Cal

Day 10 – 1200 Calorie Meal Plan

BREAKFAST	Calories	Totals
Orange juice (½ cup)	50	
Wild blueberry pancakes (Day 10 Recipe - page 86)	190	
Light syrup (1½ Tbsp)	45	
Coffee	10	295 Cal
SNACK		
Coffee or tea	10	10 Cal
LUNCH		
Peanut butter (2 Tbsp) on 2 slices of whole-grain bread	330	
Skim milk (4 oz)	45	
Fresh fruit in season (apple, plum, etc)	70	445 Cal
SNACK		
Coffee or tea	10	10 Cal
DINNER		
Broiled pork chop (about ½" thick & trimmed of fat)	260	
Green peas (½ cup)	55	
Tomato & cucumbers salad with 1 Tbsp dressing	105	
Water with lemon wedge	10	430Cal
SNACK		
Coffee or tea	10	10 Cal
		1200 Cal

Day 11 – 1200 Calorie Meal Plan

BREAKFAST	Calories	Totals
Fresh sliced orange	75	
Cheerios (1 cup) + ½ cup skim milk + about 15 raisins	190	
Coffee	10	275 Cal
SNACK		
Fresh fruit in season (apple, plum, etc)	70	70 Cal
LUNCH		
Subway 6" (Salami, Cheese + veggies)*	260	
Water or diet soda	0	260 Cal
SNACK		
Handful unsalted mixed nuts	100	100 Cal
DINNER		
Grilled chicken sausage (2 links about 2½ oz per link)	180	
Artichoke-bean salad (Day 11 Recipe - page 87)	190	
Green beans - steamed	25	
Glass of red wine (4 oz)	100	495 Cal
SNACK		
Coffee or tea	10	10 Cal
		1210 Cal

Day 12 – 1200 Calorie Meal Plan

BREAKFAST	Calories	Totals
Grapefruit (½)	75	
Scrambled egg	80	
Whole-grain toast (1 slice)	65	
Coffee	10	230 Cal
SNACK		
Coffee or tea	10	10 Cal
LUNCH		
Soup (Appendix C - **page 114**)*	140	
Tomato slices, ¼ cup chopped fresh basil + ½ tsp Evoo	40	
Whole-grain bread (1 slice)	65	
Hot or iced tea	10	265 Cal
* 30 calories added to account for flavor enhancements.		
SNACK		
Greek Yogurt (6 oz, nonfat, any flavor)	90	90 Cal
DINNER		
Eat Out – Fish dinner (Day 12 Recipe - page 88)	495	
Glass red wine (4 oz)	100	595 Cal
SNACK		
Coffee or tea	10	10 Cal
		1200 Cal

Day 13 – 1200 Calorie Meal Plan

BREAKFAST	Calories	Totals
Orange juice (½ cup)	50	
Shredded Wheat (1 cup) + ½ cup skim milk + ½ banana	260	
Coffee	10	320 Cal
SNACK		
Coffee or tea	10	10 Cal
LUNCH		
Turkey frank (2 oz) with mustard & relish	150	
Hot dog bun	125	
Water or diet soda	0	275 Cal
SNACK		
Fresh fruit in season (pear, plum, etc)	70	70 Cal
DINNER		
Pasta with Marinara sauce (Day 13 Recipe - page 89)	225	
Large salad with 2 Tbsp dressing	150	
Italian or French bread (1 slice)	80	
Water	0	455 Cal
SNACK		
Fiber One Chocolate Fudge Brownie	90	90 Cal
		1220 Cal

Day 14 – 1200 Calorie Meal Plan

BREAKFAST	Calories	Totals
Cantaloupe (½ medium)	50	
Oatena cereal mix (Day 14 Recipe - page 90)	310	
Coffee	10	370 Cal
SNACK		
Coffee or tea	10	10 Cal
LUNCH		
Grilled Swiss cheese sandwich (2 oz low-fat cheese)	310	
Diet soda or water	0	310 Cal
SNACK		
Small bunch of grapes	65	65 Cal
DINNER		
Frozen chicken dinner (Day 28 Recipe - page 104)	300	
Small salad with 1 Tbsp dressing	75	
Water	0	375 Cal
SNACK		
Greek Yogurt (6 oz, nonfat, any flavor)	90	90 Cal
		1220 Cal

Day 15 – 1200 Calorie Meal Plan

BREAKFAST	Calories	Totals
Fresh or frozen strawberries (1 cup)	50	
French toast (made with 2 slices whole-grain bread)	250	
Light syrup (1 Tbsp)	30	
Coffee	10	340 Cal
SNACK		
Coffee or tea	10	10 Cal
LUNCH		
Salad (3 oz tuna, 1 tsp Evoo, onions & celery)	175	
Lettuce & tomato wedges	20	
Rye bread (1 slice)	65	
Coffee or tea	10	270 Cal
SNACK		
Greek Yogurt (6 oz, nonfat, any flavor)	90	
Coffee or tea	10	100 Cal
DINNER		
London broil (Day 15 Recipe - page 91)	320	
Brown rice (½ cup)	100	
Broccoli (1 cup steamed)	50	
Water	0	470 Cal
SNACK		
Coffee or tea	10	10 Cal
		1200 Cal

Day 16 – 1200 Calorie Meal Plan

BREAKFAST	Calories	Totals
Orange juice (½ cup)	50	
Wheat Chex (¾ cup) + ½ cup skim milk + ½ banana	250	
Coffee	10	310 Cal
SNACK		
Coffee or tea	10	10 Cal
LUNCH		
Subway 6" (Roast Beef, Cheese + veggies)	245	
Diet soda or water	0	245 Cal
SNACK		
Fresh fruit in season (apple, peach, etc)	70	
Coffee or tea	10	80 Cal
DINNER		
Baked red snapper (Day 16 Recipe - page 92)	215	
Wild rice mix	160	
Green beans & tomato	75	
Water with lemon section	10	460 Cal
SNACK		
Greek Yogurt (6 oz, nonfat, any flavor)	90	
Coffee or tea	10	100 Cal
		1195 Cal

Day 17 – 1200 Calorie Meal Plan

BREAKFAST	Calories	Totals
Cantaloupe (½ medium)	50	
Fried egg	80	
Turkey bacon (1 slice)	35	
Toasted raisin bread (1 slice)	75	
Coffee	10	250 Cal
SNACK		
Coffee or tea	10	10 Cal
LUNCH		
Soup (Appendix C - page 114)	160	
Lettuce & tomato sandwich with Tbsp light mayo	170	
Cucumber slices and carrot & celery sticks	15	
Hot or iced tea	10	355 Cal
SNACK		
Greek Yogurt (6 oz, nonfat, any flavor)	90	90 Cal
DINNER		
Cajun chicken salad (Day 17 Recipe - page 93)	330	
Whole-grain bread (1 slice)	65	
Fresh fruit in season (pear, plum, etc)	70	
Water with lemon section	10	475 Cal
SNACK		
Coffee or tea	10	10 Cal
		1190 Cal

Day 18 – 1200 Calorie Meal Plan

BREAKFAST	Calories	Totals
Grapefruit (½)	75	
Cheerios (1 cup) + ½ cup skim milk + about 15 raisins	190	
Coffee	10	275 Cal
SNACK		
Coffee or tea	10	10 Cal
LUNCH		
Cottage cheese (1 cup low fat)	180	
Small salad with 1 Tbsp low-cal dressing	75	
Hot or iced tea	10	265 Cal
SNACK		
Handful unsalted mixed nuts	100	100 Cal
DINNER		
Grilled swordfish (Day 18 Recipe - page 94)	250	
Grilled potatoes	100	
Grilled cherry tomatoes	40	
Spinach (½ cup) steamed with garlic & drizzled Evoo	50	
Glass of red wine (4 oz)	100	540 Cal
SNACK		
Coffee or tea	10	10 Cal
		1200 Cal

Day 19 – 1200 Calorie Meal Plan

BREAKFAST	Calories	Totals
Grapefruit (½)	75	
Scrambled egg	80	
Whole-grain toast (1 slice)	65	
Coffee	10	230 Cal
SNACK		
Coffee or tea	10	10 Cal
LUNCH		
Soup (Appendix C - page 114)	180	
Turkey (1 oz) on 1 slice of rye bread (½ sandwich)	115	
Hot or iced tea	10	305 Cal
SNACK		
Coffee or tea	10	10 Cal
DINNER		
Eat Out – Italian food (Day 19 Recipe - page 95)	540	
Glass red wine (4 oz)	100	640 Cal
SNACK		
Coffee or tea	10	10 Cal
		1205 Cal

Day 20 – 1200 Calorie Meal Plan

BREAKFAST	Calories	Totals
Tomato juice (½ cup)	20	
Shredded Wheat (1 cup) + ½ cup skim milk	210	
Coffee	10	240 Cal
SNACK		
Handful unsalted mixed nuts	100	100 Cal
LUNCH		
Left over Italian food from Day 19	260	
Hot or iced tea	10	270 Cal
SNACK		
Greek Yogurt (6 oz, nonfat, any flavor)	90	90 Cal
DINNER		
Spaghetti alla Puttanesca (Day 20 Recipe - page 96)	345	
Large salad with 2 Tbsp dressing	150	
Water	0	495 Cal
SNACK		
Coffee or tea	10	10 Cal
		1205 Cal

Day 21 – 1200 Calorie Meal Plan

BREAKFAST	Calories	Totals
Cantaloupe (½ medium)	50	
Oatmeal (½ cup dry) + ½ cup skim milk + about 15 raisins	220	
Coffee	10	280 Cal
SNACK		
Coffee or tea	10	10 Cal
LUNCH		
Turkey breast (2 oz) sandwich	235	
Lettuce & tomato with Tbsp light mayo	35	
Fresh fruit in season (apple, plum, etc)	70	
Water	0	340 Cal
SNACK		
Coffee or tea	10	10 Cal
DINNER		
Frozen meat dinner (Day 21 Recipe - page 97)	300	
Large salad with 2 Tbsp dressing	150	
Glass red wine (4 oz)	100	550 Cal
SNACK		
Coffee or tea	10	10 Cal
		1200 Cal

Day 22 – 1200 Calorie Meal Plan

BREAKFAST	Calories	Totals
Fresh or frozen strawberries (1 cup)	25	
French toasted English Muffin (Day 2 Recipe - page 78)	270	
Light syrup (1 Tbsp)	30	
Coffee	10	335 Cal
SNACK		
Coffee or tea	10	10 Cal
LUNCH		
Salad (3 oz tuna, 1 tsp Evoo, onions & celery)	175	
Lettuce & tomato wedges	20	
Italian or French bread (1 slice - see page 8)	80	
Hot or iced tea	10	285 Cal
SNACK		
Coffee or tea	10	10 Cal
DINNER		
Shrimp & spinach salad (Day 22 Recipe page 98)	310	
Italian or French bread (1 slice)	80	
Large salad with 2 Tbsp dressing	150	
Water with lemon section	10	550 Cal
SNACK		
Coffee or tea	10	10 Cal
		1200 Cal

Day 23 – 1200 Calorie Meal Plan

BREAKFAST	Calories	Totals
Cantaloupe (½ medium)	50	
Wheaties (¾ cup) + ½ cup skim milk + ½ banana	190	
Whole-grain toast (1 slice)	65	
Coffee	10	315 Cal
SNACK		
Coffee or tea	10	10 Cal
LUNCH		
Ham (2 oz) with mustard on 2 slices rye bread	290	
Lettuce & tomato wedges	20	
Water or diet soda	0	310 Cal
SNACK		
Handful unsalted mixed nuts	100	
Coffee or tea	10	110 Cal
DINNER		
Beans & greens salad (Day 23 Recipe - page 99)	260	
Baked potato (medium)	100	
Hot or iced tea	10	370 Cal
SNACK		
Fresh fruit in season (apple, peach, etc)	70	70 Cal
		1195 Cal

Day 24 – 1200 Calorie Meal Plan

BREAKFAST	Calories	Totals
Fresh orange sliced	75	
Soft-boiled egg	80	
Whole-grain toast (1 slice)	65	
Coffee	10	230 Cal
SNACK		
Greek Yogurt (6 oz, nonfat, any flavor)	90	90 Cal
LUNCH		
Salad – 3 oz salmon, 1 tsp Evoo, onions & celery	200	
Lettuce & tomato wedges	20	
Rye bread (1 slice)	65	
Coffee or tea	10	295 Cal
SNACK		
Coffee or tea	10	10 Cal
DINNER		
Chicken breast – broiled (5 oz)	240	
Four bean plus salad (½ cup) (Day 24 Recipe page 100)	135	
Large salad with 2 Tbsp dressing	150	
Water	0	525 Cal
SNACK		
Fresh fruit in season (pear, plum, etc)	70	70 Cal
		1220 Cal

Day 25 – 1200 Calorie Meal Plan

BREAKFAST	Calories	Totals
Grapefruit (½)	75	
Cheerios (1 cup) + ½ cup skim milk + about 15 raisins	190	
Coffee	10	275 Cal
SNACK		
Coffee or tea	10	10 Cal
LUNCH		
Subway 6" (Ham, Cheese + veggies)	260	
Diet soda or water	0	260 Cal
SNACK		
Fresh fruit in season (peach, plum, etc)	70	
Coffee or tea	10	80 Cal
DINNER		
Hanger steak (Day 25 Recipe - page 101)	320	
Roasted potatoes (Day 25 Recipe)	120	
Cherry tomatoes (Day 25 Recipe)	20	
Steamed spinach (½ cup)	25	
Glass red wine (4 oz)	100	585 Cal
SNACK		
Coffee or tea	10	10 Cal
		1220 Cal

Day 26 – 1200 Calorie Meal Plan

BREAKFAST	Calories	Totals
Cantaloupe (½ medium)	50	
Fried egg	80	
Toasted whole-grain bread (1 slice)	65	
Coffee	10	205 Cal
SNACK		
Greek Yogurt (6 oz, nonfat, any flavor)	90	90 Cal
LUNCH		
Soup (Appendix C - page 114)	200	
Italian or French bread (1 slice)	80	
Lettuce & tomato slices	20	
Hot or iced tea	10	310 Cal
SNACK		
Fresh fruit in season (apple, plum, etc)	70	
Coffee or tea	10	80 Cal
DINNER		
Grilled scallops (Day 26 Recipe - page 102)	210	
Grilled polenta (Day 26 Recipe)	125	
Mushroom-steamed green beans-red onion	45	
Grilled asparagus	10	
Water	0	390 Cal
SNACK		
Popcorn Mini Bag	110	
Coffee or tea	10	120 Cal
		1195 Cal

Day 27 – 1200 Calorie Meal Plan

BREAKFAST	Calories	Totals
Cantaloupe (½ medium)	50	
Oatmeal (½ cup dry) + ½ cup skim milk + 15 raisins	220	
Coffee	10	280 Cal
SNACK		
Fresh fruit in season (pear, plum, etc)	70	70 Cal
LUNCH		
Two servings (1 cup) left over Day 24 bean salad	270	
Italian or French bread (1 slice)	80	
Lettuce & tomato slices	20	
Water	0	370 Cal
SNACK		
Coffee or tea	10	10 Cal
DINNER		
Fettuccine (Day 27 Recipe - page 103)	290	
Small salad with 1 Tbsp dressing	75	
Glass red wine (4 oz)	100	465 Cal
SNACK		
Coffee or tea	10	10 Cal
		1205 Cal

Day 28 – 1200 Calorie Meal Plan

BREAKFAST	Calories	Totals
Tomato juice (½ cup)	20	
Shredded Wheat (1 cup) + ½ cup skim milk + ½ banana	260	
Coffee	10	290 Cal
SNACK		
Coffee or tea	10	10 Cal
LUNCH		
Roast beef sandwich (2 oz) on whole-grain bread	295	
Lettuce	0	
Fresh fruit in season (peach, plum, etc)	70	
Hot or iced tea	10	375 Cal
SNACK		
Handful unsalted mixed nuts	100	100 Cal
DINNER		
Frozen chicken dinner (Day 28 Recipe - page 104)	300	
Large salad with 2 Tbsp dressing	150	
Water	0	435 Cal
SNACK		
Coffee or tea	10	10 Cal
		1210 Cal

Day 29 – 1200 Calorie Meal Plan

BREAKFAST	Calories	Totals
Orange juice (½ cup)	50	
Wild blueberry pancakes (Day 10 Recipe - page 85)	190	
Turkey bacon (1 slice)	35	
Light syrup (1 Tbsp)	30	
Coffee	10	315 Cal
SNACK		
Greek Yogurt (6 oz, nonfat, any flavor)	90	
Coffee or tea	10	100 Cal
LUNCH		
Salad (3 oz tuna, 1 tsp Evoo, onions & celery)	175	
Lettuce & tomato wedges	20	
Italian or French bread	80	
Hot or ice tea	10	285 Cal
SNACK		
Coffee or tea	10	10 Cal
DINNER		
Barbequed shrimp (Day 29 Recipe - page 105)	160	
Corn on the cob (medium)	100	
Steamed broccoli (1 cup equivalent)	50	
Glass red wine (4 oz)	100	410 Cal
SNACK		
Fresh fruit in season (apple, peach, etc)	70	
Coffee or tea	10	80 Cal
		1200 Cal

Day 30 – 1200 Calorie Meal Plan

BREAKFAST	Calories	Totals
Fresh orange sliced	75	
Wheat Chex (¾ cup) + ½ cup skim milk + ½ banana	250	
Coffee	10	335 Cal
SNACK		
Coffee or tea	10	10 Cal
LUNCH		
Soup (Appendix C - page 114)	170	
Italian or French bread (1 slice)	80	
Raw zucchini slices, celery & carrot sticks	20	
Hot or iced tea	10	280 Cal
SNACK		
Coffee or tea	10	10 Cal
DINNER		
Pasta e Fagioli (Day 30 Recipe - page 106)	300	
Small salad with 1 Tbsp dressing	75	
Italian or French bread (1 slice)	80	
Glass red wine (4 oz)	100	555 Cal
SNACK		
Coffee or tea	10	10 Cal
		1200 Cal

1500-Calorie
Daily Menus

Day 1 – 1500 Calorie Meal Plan

BREAKFAST	Calories	Totals
Grapefruit (½)	75	
Scrambled egg (See **Notes** - page 12)	80	
Turkey bacon (2 slices)	70	
Whole grain toast (1 slice) (see page 9)	65	
Coffee (see page 12)	10	300 Cal
SNACK		
Greek Yogurt (6 oz, plain, nonfat)	90	90 Cal
LUNCH		
Ham (2 oz) with mustard on 2 slices rye bread	290	
Small bunch of grapes	65	
Hot or iced tea	10	365 Cal
SNACK		
Handful unsalted mixed nuts	100	100 Cal
DINNER		
Chicken w Peppers & Onions (Day 1 Recipe - page 77)	250	
Remaining food - Day 1 Recipe	70	
Whole-grain bread (1 slice)	65	
Large salad with 2 Tbsp dressing (see page 9)	150	
Glass red wine (4 oz)	100	
Water	0	635 Cal
SNACK		
Coffee or tea	10	10 Cal
		1500 Cal

Day 2 – 1500 Calorie Meal Plan

BREAKFAST	Calories	Totals
Fresh or frozen strawberries (½ cup)	25	
French toasted English Muffin (Day 2 Recipe - page 78)	270	
Light syrup (1 Tbsp)	30	
Coffee (See **Notes** - page 12)	10	335 Cal
SNACK		
Greek Yogurt (6 oz, plain, nonfat)	90	90 Cal
LUNCH		
Salad (3 oz tuna, 1 tsp Evoo, onions & celery)	175	
Italian or French bread (1 slice - see page 9)	80	
Fresh fruit in season (apple, plum, etc)	70	
Water	0	325 Cal
SNACK		
Handful unsalted mixed nuts	100	100 Cal
DINNER		
Broiled veal chop (4 oz lean)	200	
Corn on the cob (1 medium ear)	100	
Broccoli (½ cup steamed)	30	
Large salad with 2 Tbsp dressing	150	
Glass red wine (4 oz)	100	580 Cal
SNACK		
Graham crackers (2 squares)	60	
Coffee or tea	10	70 Cal
		1500 Cal

Day 3 – 1500 Calorie Meal Plan

BREAKFAST	Calories	Totals
Orange juice (½ cup)	50	
Wheaties (¾ cup) + ½ cup skim milk + ½ banana	190	
Whole-grain toast (1 slice) (See page 8)	65	
Coffee	10	315 Cal
SNACK		
Fresh fruit in season (apple, peach, etc)	70	70 Cal
LUNCH		
Soup (Appendix C - page 114)*	110	
Turkey breast (1 oz) on 1 slice rye bread	105	
Lettuce & tomato slices	20	
Diet soda or water	0	235 Cal
* 30 calories added to account for flavor enhancements.		
SNACK		
Two small cookies -Oatmeal, ginger, etc. Check calories!	160	
Coffee or tea	10	170 Cal
DINNER		
Baked Herb-Crusted Cod (Day 3 Recipe - page 79)	230	
Spinach (½ cup) steamed with garlic & drizzled	100	
Asparagus (7 spear cooked & drained)	20	
Baked potato (medium)	100	
Italian or French bread (1 slice)	80	
Glass red wine (4 oz)	100	630 Cal
SNACK		
Fiber One Chocolate Fudge Brownie	90	90 Cal
		1510 Cal

Day 4 – 1500 Calorie Meal Plan

BREAKFAST	Calories	Totals
Grapefruit (½)	75	
Cheerios (1 cup) + ½ cup skim milk + about 15 raisins*	190	
Coffee	10	275 Cal
SNACK		
Fresh fruit in season (apple, peach, etc)	70	70 Cal
LUNCH		
Cottage cheese (1 cup low fat)	180	
Large salad with 2 Tbsp dressing	150	
Hot or iced tea	10	340 Cal
SNACK		
Handful unsalted mixed nuts	100	100 Cal
DINNER		
Pasta and Veggies (Day 4 Recipe - page 80)	460	
Italian or French bread (1 slice)	80	
Glass red wine (4 oz)	100	640 Cal
SNACK		
One small cookie	80	
Coffee or tea	10	90 Cal
* See **Notes** - page 11 re substituting blueberries for raisins.		1515 Cal

Day 5 – 1500 Calorie Meal Plan

BREAKFAST	Calories	Totals
Cantaloupe (½ medium)	50	
Fried egg	80	
Toasted raisin bread (1 slice)	75	
Coffee	10	215 Cal
SNACK		
Greek Yogurt (6 oz, nonfat, any flavor)	90	
Coffee or tea	10	100 Cal
LUNCH		
Soup (Appendix C - page 114)	150	
Italian or French bread (1 slice)	80	
Lettuce and sliced tomato with 1 Tbsp dressing	85	
Hot or iced tea	10	325 Cal
* 30 calories added to account for flavor enhancements.		
SNACK		
Popcorn Mini Bag	110	
Coffee or tea	10	120 Cal
DINNER		
Frozen fish dinner (Day 5 Recipe - page 81)	340	
Large salad with 2 Tbsp dressing	150	
Italian or French bread (1 slice)	80	
Glass red wine (4 oz)	100	670 Cal
SNACK		
Fresh fruit in season (apple, peach, etc)	70	70 Cal
		1500 Cal

Day 6 – 1500 Calorie Meal Plan

BREAKFAST	Calories	Totals
Tomato juice (½ cup)	20	
Shredded Wheat (1 cup) + ½ cup skim milk + ½ banana	265	
Coffee	10	295 Cal
SNACK		
Handful unsalted mixed nuts	100	
Coffee or tea	10	110 Cal
LUNCH		
Ham (2 oz) with mustard on 2 slices rye bread	290	
Lettuce	10	
Hot or iced tea	10	310 Cal
SNACK		
Greek Yogurt (6 oz, nonfat, any flavor)	90	
Coffee or tea	10	100 Cal
DINNER		
Pizza (Day 6 Recipe - page 82)	350	
Large salad with 2 Tbsp dressing	150	
Glass of red wine (4 oz)	100	
Fresh fruit in season (peach, plum, etc)	70	
Water with lemon wedge	10	670 Cal
SNACK		
Coffee or tea	10	10 Cal
		1495 Cal

Day 7 – 1500 Calorie Meal Plan

BREAKFAST	Calories	Totals
Cantaloupe (½ medium)	50	
Oatmeal (½ cup dry) + ½ cup skim milk + about 15 raisins	220	
Coffee	10	280 Cal
SNACK		
Fresh fruit in season (pear, plum, etc)	70	70 Cal
LUNCH		
Soup (Appendix C - page 114)	120	
Grilled cheese sandwich (2 slices 2% cheese)	230	
Lettuce and sliced tomato	20	
Water	0	370 Cal
SNACK		
Carrot sticks + ¼ cup low-fat cottage cheese & chives	60	60 Cal
DINNER		
Eat Out – Chicken dinner (Day 7 Recipe - page 83)	530	
Glass red wine (4 oz)	100	630 Cal
SNACK		
Graham crackers (3 squares)	90	
Coffee or tea	10	100 Cal
		1510 Cal

Day 8 – 1500 Calorie Meal Plan

BREAKFAST	Calories	Totals
Cantaloupe (½ medium)	50	
Wheaties (¾ cup) + ½ cup skim milk + ½ banana	190	
Whole-grain toast (1 slice)	65	
Coffee	10	315 Cal
SNACK		
Fresh fruit in season (apple, peach, etc)	70	70 Cal
LUNCH		
Soup (Appendix C - page 114)	160	
Turkey (1 oz) on 1 slice of rye bread (½ sandwich)	115	
Lettuce & tomato slices	20	
Hot or iced tea	10	305 Cal
SNACK		
Two small cookies	160	
Coffee or tea	10	170 Cal
DINNER		
Baked salmon with salsa (Day 8 Recipe - page 84)	215	
Summer squash, zucchini and tomatoes	60	
Brown rice (½ cup)	100	
Large salad with 2 Tbsp dressing	150	
Glass red wine (4 oz)	100	625 Cal
SNACK		
Coffee or tea	10	10 Cal
		1495 Cal

Day 9 – 1500 Calorie Meal Plan

BREAKFAST	Calories	Totals
Orange juice (½ cup)	50	
Soft-boiled (or poached) egg	80	
Whole-grain toast (2 slices)	130	
Coffee	10	270 Cal
SNACK		
Greek Yogurt (6 oz, nonfat, any flavor)	90	90 Cal
LUNCH		
Tuna salad (3 oz tuna, 1 tsp Evoo, onions & celery)	175	
Lettuce & tomato wedges + rye bread (1 slice)	85	
Fresh fruit in season – (apple, pear, etc)	70	
Coffee or tea	10	340 Cal
SNACK		
Handful unsalted mixed nuts	100	100 Cal
DINNER		
Veggie burger – (1 patty) (Day 9 Recipe - page 85)	100	
Low-fat cheddar cheese (1 thin slice)	50	
Beets (3 small) + Seeded hamburger roll	185	
Large salad with 2 Tbsp dressing	150	
Glass red wine (4 oz)	100	585 Cal
SNACK		
Graham crackers (4 squares)	120	
Coffee or tea	10	130 Cal
		1515 Cal

Day 10 – 1500 Calorie Meal Plan

BREAKFAST	Calories	Totals
Orange juice (½ cup)	50	
Wild blueberry pancakes (Day 10 Recipe - page 86)	190	
Turkey bacon (2 slices)	70	
Light syrup (1½ Tbsp)	45	
Coffee	10	365 Cal
SNACK		
Greek Yogurt (6 oz, nonfat, any flavor)	90	90 Cal
LUNCH		
Peanut butter (2 Tbsp) on 2 slices of whole-grain bread	330	
Skim milk (4 oz)	45	
Fresh fruit in season (apple, peach, etc)	70	445 Cal
SNACK		
Handful unsalted mixed nuts	100	
Coffee or tea	10	110 Cal
DINNER		
Broiled pork chop (about ½" thick trimmed of fat)	260	
Green peas (½ cup)	55	
Tomato & cucumber salad with 1 Tbsp dressing	75	
Water	0	390 Cal
SNACK		
Fiber One Chocolate Fudge Brownie	90	
Coffee or tea	10	100 Cal
		1500 Cal

Day 11 – 1500 Calorie Meal Plan

BREAKFAST	Calories	Totals
Fresh sliced orange	75	
Cheerios (1 cup) + ½ cup skim milk + about 15 raisins	190	
Whole grain toast (1 slice)	65	
Coffee	10	340 Cal
SNACK		
Fresh fruit in season (pear, plum, etc)	70	70 Cal
LUNCH		
Cottage cheese (1 cup low fat)	180	
Large salad with 2 Tbsp dressing	150	
Hot or iced tea	10	340 Cal
SNACK		
Handful unsalted mixed nuts	100	
Coffee or tea	10	110 Cal
DINNER		
Grilled chicken sausage (2 links about 2½ oz per link)	180	
Artichoke-bean salad (Day 11 Recipe - page 87)	190	
Green beans - steamed	25	
Italian or French bread (1 slice)	80	
Water with lemon wedge	10	470 Cal
SNACK		
Two small cookies	160	
Coffee or tea	10	170 Cal
		1500 Cal

Day 12 – 1500 Calorie Meal Plan

BREAKFAST	Calories	Totals
Grapefruit (½)	75	
Scrambled egg	80	
Turkey bacon (2 slices)	70	
Whole-grain toast (1 slice)	65	
Coffee	10	300 Cal
SNACK		
Greek Yogurt (6 oz, nonfat, any flavor)	90	90 Cal
LUNCH		
Soup (Appendix C - page 114)	150	
Tomato slices (¼ cup chopped fresh basil + 1 tsp Evoo)	60	
Italian or French bread (1 slice)	80	
Hot or iced tea	10	300 Cal
SNACK		
Fresh fruit in season (apple, plum, etc)	70	
Coffee or tea	10	80 Cal
DINNER		
Eat Out – Fish dinner (Day 12 Recipe - page 88)	495	
Glass red wine (4 oz)	100	595 Cal
SNACK		
Graham crackers (4 squares)	120	
Coffee or tea	10	130 Cal
		1495 Cal

Day 13 – 1500 Calorie Meal Plan

BREAKFAST	Calories	Totals
Orange juice (½ cup)	50	
Shredded Wheat (1 cup) + ½ cup skim milk + ½ banana	260	
Coffee	10	320 Cal
SNACK		
Handful unsalted mixed nuts	100	100 Cal
LUNCH		
Turkey frank (2 oz) with mustard & relish	150	
Hot dog bun	130	
Diet soda or water	0	280 Cal
SNACK		
Greek Yogurt (6 oz, nonfat, any flavor)	90	
Coffee or tea	10	100 Cal
DINNER		
Pasta - Marinara sauce (Day 13 Recipe - page 89)	225	
Large green salad with 1½ Tbsp low-cal dressing	70	
Fresh fruit in season (apple, plum, etc)	70	
Italian or French bread (1 slice)	80	
Glass of red wine (4 oz)	100	
Water with lemon wedge	10	555 Cal
SNACK		
Graham crackers (4 squares)	120	
Coffee or tea	10	130 Cal
		1485 Cal

Day 14 – 1500 Calorie Meal Plan

BREAKFAST	Calories	Totals
Cantaloupe (½ medium)	50	
Oatena cereal mix (Day 14 Recipe - page 90)	310	
Whole-grain toast (1 slice)	65	
Coffee	10	435 Cal
SNACK		
Fresh fruit in season (peach, plum, etc)	70	
Coffee or tea	10	80 Cal
LUNCH		
Grilled Swiss cheese sandwich (2 oz low-fat cheese)	310	
Hot or iced tea	10	320 Cal
SNACK		
Handful unsalted mixed nuts	100	
Coffee or tea	10	110 Cal
DINNER		
Frozen chicken dinner (Day 28 Recipe - page 104)	300	
Small salad with 1 Tbsp dressing	75	
Water with lemon wedge	10	385 Cal
SNACK		
Dark chocolate (1 oz)	150	
Coffee or tea	10	160 Cal
		1490 Cal

Day 15 – 1500 Calorie Meal Plan

BREAKFAST	Calories	Totals
Fresh or frozen strawberries (1 cup)	50	
French toast (2 slices whole-grain bread)	250	
Light syrup (1 Tbsp)	30	
Coffee	10	340 Cal
SNACK		
Greek Yogurt (6 oz, nonfat, any flavor)	90	90 Cal
LUNCH		
Tuna salad (3 oz tuna, 1 tsp Evoo, onions & celery)	175	
Lettuce & tomato wedges	20	
Italian or French bread (1 slice)	80	
Hot or ice tea	10	285 Cal
SNACK		
Handful unsalted mixed nuts	100	
Coffee or tea	10	110 Cal
DINNER		
London broil (Day 15 Recipe - page 91)	320	
Brown rice (½ cup)	100	
Broccoli (1 cup steamed)	50	
Fresh fruit in season (apple, plum, etc)	70	
Water with lemon wedge	10	550 Cal
SNACK		
Graham crackers (4 squares)	120	
Coffee or tea	10	130 Cal
		1505 Cal

Day 16 – 1500 Calorie Meal Plan

BREAKFAST	Calories	Totals
Orange juice (½ cup)	50	
Wheat Chex (¾ cup) + ½ cup skim milk + ½ banana	250	
Coffee	10	310 Cal
SNACK		
Handful unsalted mixed nuts	100	
Coffee or tea	10	110 Cal
LUNCH		
Subway 6" (Roast Beef, Cheese + veggies)	245	
Fresh fruit in season (peach, plum, etc)	70	
Hot or ice tea	10	325 Cal
SNACK		
Coffee or tea	10	10 Cal
DINNER		
Baked red snapper (Day 16 Recipe - page 92)	215	
Wild rice mix	160	
Green beans & tomato	75	
Italian or French bread (1 slice)	80	
Glass red wine (4 oz)	100	630 Cal
SNACK		
Fiber One Chocolate Fudge Brownie	90	
Coffee or tea	10	100 Cal
		1485 Cal

Day 17 – 1500 Calorie Meal Plan

BREAKFAST	Calories	Totals
Cantaloupe (½ medium)	50	
Fried egg	80	
Turkey bacon (2 slices)	70	
Toasted raisin bread (1 slice)	75	
Coffee	10	285 Cal
SNACK		
Greek Yogurt (6 oz, nonfat, any flavor)	90	90 Cal
LUNCH		
Soup (Appendix C - page 114)	170	
Lettuce & tomato sandwich (tsp light mayonnaise)	170	
Cucumber slices and carrots and celery sticks	15	
Hot or iced tea	10	365 Cal
SNACK		
Handful unsalted mixed nuts	100	
Coffee or tea	10	110 Cal
DINNER		
Cajun chicken salad (Day 17 Recipe - page 93)	330	
Italian or French bread (1 slice)	80	
Fresh fruit in season (apple, peach, etc)	70	
Water with lemon wedge	10	490 Cal
SNACK		
Dark chocolate (1 oz)	150	
Coffee or tea	10	160 Cal
		1500 Cal

Day 18 – 1500 Calorie Meal Plan

BREAKFAST	Calories	Totals
Grapefruit (½)	75	
Cheerios (1 cup) + ½ cup skim milk + about 15 raisins	190	
Coffee	10	275 Cal
SNACK		
Fresh fruit in season (peach, plum, etc)	70	
Coffee or tea	10	80 Cal
LUNCH		
Cottage cheese (1 cup low fat)	180	
Large salad with 2 Tbsp dressing	150	
Hot or iced tea	10	340 Cal
SNACK		
Handful unsalted mixed nuts	100	
Coffee or tea	10	110 Cal
DINNER		
Grilled swordfish (Day 18 Recipe - page 94)	250	
Grilled potatoes	100	
Grilled cherry tomatoes	45	
Spinach (½ cup) steamed w garlic & drizzled Evoo	50	
Italian or French bread (1 slice)	80	
Water	0	525 Cal
SNACK		
Two small cookies	160	
Coffee or tea	10	170 Cal
		1500 Cal

Day 19 – 1500 Calorie Meal Plan

BREAKFAST	Calories	Totals
Grapefruit (½)	75	
Scrambled egg	80	
Whole grain toast (2 slices)	130	
Coffee	10	295 Cal
SNACK		
Yogurt (6 oz, nonfat, any flavor)	90	90 Cal
LUNCH		
Soup (Appendix C - page 114)	120	
Turkey (1 oz) on 1 slice of rye bread	115	
Lettuce & tomato slices	20	
Hot or iced tea	10	265 Cal
SNACK		
Fresh fruit in season (apple, plum, etc)	70	70 Cal
DINNER		
Eat Out – Italian food (Day 19 Recipe - page 95)	540	
Glass red wine (4 oz)	100	640 Cal
SNACK		
Graham crackers (3 squares)	90	
Skim milk (4 oz)	45	165 Cal
		1495 Cal

Day 20 – 1500 Calorie Meal Plan

BREAKFAST	Calories	Totals
Tomato juice (½ cup)	20	
Shredded Wheat (1 cup) + ½ cup skim milk + ½ banana	260	
Coffee	10	290 Cal
SNACK		
Handful unsalted mixed nuts	100	100 Cal
LUNCH		
Left over Italian food from Day 19	260	
Hot or iced tea	10	270 Cal
SNACK		
Greek Yogurt (6 oz, nonfat, any flavor)	90	
Coffee or tea	10	100 Cal
DINNER		
Spaghetti alla Puttanesca (Day 20 Recipe - page 96)	345	
Small salad with 1 Tbsp dressing	75	
Italian or French bread (1 slice)	80	
Glass of red wine (4 oz)	100	
Water with lemon wedge	10	610 Cal
SNACK		
Graham crackers (4 squares)	120	
Coffee or tea	10	130 Cal
		1500 Cal

Day 21 – 1500 Calorie Meal Plan

BREAKFAST	Calories	Totals
Cantaloupe (½ medium)	50	
Oatmeal (½ cup dry) + ½ cup skim milk + about 15 raisins	220	
Coffee	10	280 Cal
SNACK		
Handful unsalted mixed nuts	100	100 Cal
LUNCH		
Turkey breast (2 oz) sandwich	235	
Lettuce, tomato and tsp light mayo	35	
Fresh fruit in season (apple, plum, etc)	70	
Water	0	340 Cal
SNACK		
Greek Yogurt (6 oz, nonfat, any flavor)	90	90 Cal
DINNER		
Frozen meat dinner (Day 21 Recipe - page 97)	300	
Large salad with 2 Tbsp dressing	150	
Italian or French bread (1 slice)	80	
Glass red wine (4 oz)	100	630 Cal
SNACK		
Graham crackers (2 squares)	60	
Coffee or tea	10	70 Cal
		1510 Cal

Day 22 – 1500 Calorie Meal Plan

BREAKFAST	Calories	Totals
Fresh or frozen strawberries (½ cup)	25	
French toasted English Muffin (Day 2 Recipe - page 79)	270	
Light syrup (1 Tbsp)	30	
Coffee	10	335 Cal
SNACK		
Greek Yogurt (6 oz, nonfat, any flavor)	90	90 Cal
LUNCH		
Salad (3 oz tuna, 1 tsp Evoo, onions & celery)	175	
Lettuce & tomato wedges	20	
Italian or French bread (1 slice)	80	
Fresh fruit in season (pear, plum, etc)	70	
Diet soda or water	0	365 Cal
SNACK		
Two small cookies	160	
Coffee or tea	10	170 Cal
DINNER		
Shrimp & spinach salad (Day 22 Recipe - page 98)	310	
Italian or French bread (1 slice)	80	
Glass red wine (4 oz)	100	
Water	0	490 Cal
SNACK		
Graham crackers (2 squares)	60	
Coffee or tea	10	70 Cal
		1500 Cal

Day 23 – 1500 Calorie Meal Plan

BREAKFAST	Calories	Totals
Cantaloupe (½ medium)	50	
Wheaties (¾ cup) + ½ cup skim milk + ½ banana	190	
Whole-grain toast (1 slice)	65	
Coffee	10	315 Cal
SNACK		
Greek Yogurt (6 oz, nonfat, any flavor)	90	90 Cal
LUNCH		
Ham (2 oz) with mustard on 2 slices rye bread	290	
Small bunch of grapes	65	
Hot or iced tea	10	355 Cal
SNACK		
Handful unsalted mixed nuts	100	
Coffee or tea	10	110 Cal
DINNER		
Beans & greens salad (Day 23 Recipe - page 99)	260	
Italian or French bread (1 slice)	80	
Baked potato (medium)	100	
Fresh fruit in season (peach, plum, etc)	70	
Water	0	510 Cal
SNACK		
Graham crackers (3 squares)	90	
Coffee or tea	10	100 Cal
		1490 Cal

Day 24 – 1500 Calorie Meal Plan

BREAKFAST	Calories	Totals
Fresh orange sliced	75	
Soft-boiled egg	80	
Whole-grain toast (2 slices)	130	
Coffee	10	295 Cal
SNACK		
Handful unsalted mixed nuts	100	100 Cal
LUNCH		
Salad – 3 oz salmon, 1 tsp Evoo, onions & celery	200	
Lettuce & tomato wedges	20	
Italian or French bread (1 slice)	80	
Fresh fruit in season (apple, peach, etc)	70	
Coffee or tea	10	380 Cal
SNACK		
Popcorn Mini Bag	110	110 Cal
DINNER		
Chicken breast – broiled (5 oz)	250	
Four bean plus salad - ½ cup (Day 24 Recipe page 100)	135	
Large with 2 Tbsp dressing	150	
Italian or French bread (1 slice)	80	
Water	0	615 Cal
SNACK		
Coffee or tea	10	10 Cal
		1510 Cal

Day 25 – 1500 Calorie Meal Plan

BREAKFAST	Calories	Totals
Grapefruit (½)	75	
Cheerios (1 cup) + ½ cup skim milk + about 15 raisins	190	
Coffee	10	275 Cal
SNACK		
Fresh fruit in season (apple, peach, etc)	70	70 Cal
LUNCH		
Subway 6" (Ham, Cheese + veggies)	260	
Large salad with 2 Tbsp dressing	150	
Diet soda or water	0	410 Cal
SNACK		
Handful unsalted mixed nuts	100	100 Cal
DINNER		
Hanger steak (Day 25 Recipe - page 101)	320	
Roasted potatoes (Day 25 Recipe)	120	
Cherry tomatoes (Day 25 Recipe)	20	
Steamed spinach (½ cup)	25	
Italian or French bread (1 slice)	80	
Water	0	545 Cal
SNACK		
Graham crackers (3 squares)	90	
Coffee or tea	10	100 Cal
		1500 Cal

Day 26 – 1500 Calorie Meal Plan

BREAKFAST	Calories	Totals
Cantaloupe (½ medium)	50	
Fried egg	80	
Toasted whole-grain bread (2 slices)	130	
Coffee	10	270 Cal
SNACK		
Handful unsalted mixed nuts	100	100 Cal
LUNCH		
Soup (Appendix C - page 114)*	280	
Italian or French bread (1 slice)	80	
Lettuce & tomato slices	30	
Hot or iced tea	10	400 Cal
* Enjoy 2 servings of 140 Cal soup.		
SNACK		
Fresh fruit in season (apple, plum, etc)	70	70 Cal
DINNER		
Grilled scallops (Day 26 Recipe - page 102)	210	
Grilled polenta (Day 26 Recipe.)	125	
For preparation remaining food - see Day 26 Recipe	55	
Small salad with 1 Tbsp dressing	75	
Greek Yogurt (6 oz, nonfat, any flavor)	90	
Water with lemon wedge	10	565 Cal
SNACK		
Graham crackers (3 squares)	90	
Coffee or tea	10	100 Cal
		1505 Cal

Day 27 – 1500 Calorie Meal Plan

BREAKFAST	Calories	Totals
Cantaloupe (½ medium)	50	
Oatmeal (½ cup dry) + ½ cup skim milk + about 15 raisins	220	
Coffee	10	280 Cal
SNACK		
Fresh fruit in season (apple, plum, etc)	70	70 Cal
LUNCH		
Two servings (1 cup) left over Day 24 bean salad	270	
Small whole-grain roll	80	
Lettuce & tomato slices	20	
Hot or iced tea	10	380 Cal
SNACK		
Celery sticks + ¼ cup low-fat cottage cheese & chives	60	60 Cal
DINNER		
Fettuccine (Day 27 Recipe - page 103)	290	
Large salad with 2 Tbsp dressing	150	
Italian or French bread (1 slice)	80	
Glass of red wine (4 oz)	100	
Water	0	620 Cal
SNACK		
Fiber One Chocolate Fudge Brownie	90	
Coffee or tea	10	100 Cal
		1510 Cal

Day 28 – 1500 Calorie Meal Plan

BREAKFAST	Calories	Totals
Tomato juice (½ cup)	20	
Shredded Wheat (1 cup) + ½ cup skim milk + ½ banana	260	
Coffee	10	290 Cal
SNACK		
Handful unsalted mixed nuts	100	100 Cal
LUNCH		
Roast beef (2 oz) sandwich (whole-grain bread)	295	
Lettuce	0	
Fresh fruit in season (peach, plum, etc)	70	
Hot or iced tea	10	375 Cal
SNACK		
Greek Yogurt (6 oz, nonfat, any flavor)	90	90 Cal
DINNER		
Frozen chicken dinner (Day 28 Recipe - page 104)	300	
Large salad with 2 Tbsp dressing	150	
Italian or French bread (1 slice)	80	
Glass red wine (4 oz)	100	
Water	0	630 Cal
SNACK		
Coffee or tea	10	10 Cal
		1495 Cal

Day 29 – 1500 Calorie Meal Plan

BREAKFAST	Calories	Totals
Orange juice (½ cup)	50	
Wild blueberry pancakes (Day 10 Recipe - page 87)	190	
Turkey bacon (2 slices)	70	
Light syrup (1½ Tbsp)	45	
Coffee	10	365 Cal
SNACK		
Handful unsalted mixed nuts	100	100 Cal
LUNCH		
Salad (3 oz tuna, 1 tsp Evoo, onions & celery)	175	
Lettuce & tomato wedges	20	
Italian or French bread (1 slice)	80	
Fresh fruit in season (pear, peach, etc)	70	
Coffee or tea	10	355 Cal
SNACK		
Fiber One Chocolate Fudge Brownie	90	
Coffee or tea	10	100 Cal
DINNER		
Barbequed shrimp (Day 29 Recipe - page 105)	160	
Corn on the cob (medium)	90	
Steamed broccoli (1 cup equivalent)	60	
Greek Yogurt (6 oz, nonfat, any flavor)	90	
Water with lemon wedge	10	410 Cal
SNACK		
Two small cookies	160	
Coffee or tea	10	170 Cal
		1500 Cal

Day 30 – 1500 Calorie Meal Plan

BREAKFAST	Calories	Totals
Fresh orange sliced	75	
Wheat Chex (¾ cup) + ½ cup skim milk + ½ banana	250	
Coffee	10	335 Cal
SNACK		
Fresh fruit in season (peach, plum, etc)	70	70 Cal
LUNCH		
Soup (Appendix C - page 114)	190	
Italian or French bread (1 slice)	80	
Raw zucchini slices, celery and carrot sticks	20	
Hot or iced tea	10	300 Cal
SNACK		
Graham crackers (4 squares)	120	
Coffee or tea	10	130 Cal
DINNER		
Pasta e Fagioli (Day 30 Recipe - page 106)	300	
Small salad with 1 Tbsp dressing	75	
Italian or French bread (1 slice)	80	
Glass red wine (4 oz)	100	555 Cal
SNACK		
Handful unsalted mixed nuts	100	
Coffee or tea	10	110 Cal
		1500 Cal

Recipes & Diet Tips

Day 1 Recipe

<u>Chicken with Peppers & Onions</u>

4 boneless & skinless chicken breasts (about 5 oz each)
Coat the chicken breasts lightly with extra-virgin olive oil (EVOO).
Prepare medium-hot fire on well-oiled gas or charcoal grill . Place breasts
on grill, turning them every 4 minutes, for 10 to 12 minutes, or until done.
(To check if breasts are done, the meat should be moist and white with no
sign of pink when you cut into breast.) Serve hot.

2 medium red peppers
1 medium onion

Place peppers and onions in pan with 2 Tbsp fat-free chicken stock. Sauté
until stock is reduced. Spray pan lightly with cooking oil (see page 9) and
sauté another 2 minutes. Salt and pepper to taste.
Serves 4. About 250 Calories per serving (for chicken only).

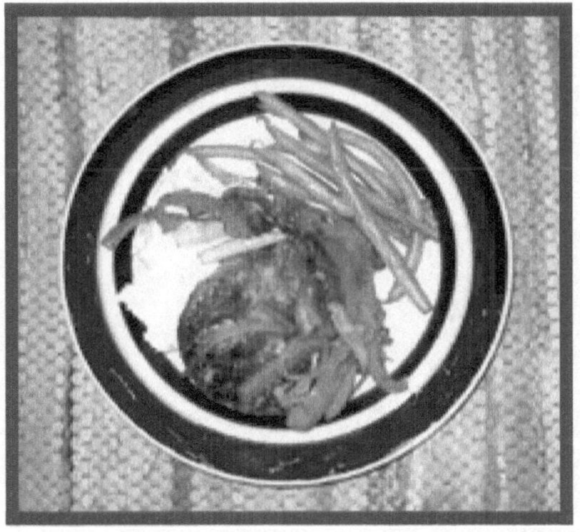

<u>Diet Tip of the Day:</u>. A **reducing diet is best supervised by a
physician**. This is especially true when a great deal of weight needs to be
lost, or if you have an ailment or a history of medical problems.

Day 2 Recipe

<u>French-Toasted English Muffin</u>

  6 whole wheat English muffins (light)
  4 eggs
  2 cups skim milk
  2 teaspoons (tsp) vanilla
  Dash of cinnamon

In a medium bowl, beat together eggs and skim milk. Add vanilla and cinnamon. Separate English muffins into halves and saturate slices in egg mixture. In a non-stick skillet coated with cooking spray (see page 9), cook muffins until both sides are golden brown. Dust lightly with confectionary sugar. Serve hot or keep in an oven or warmer at 200 ºF until ready to plate.

<u>Serves 4</u>. Three English muffin slices (1½ muffins) per serving. Serving is 270 Calories.

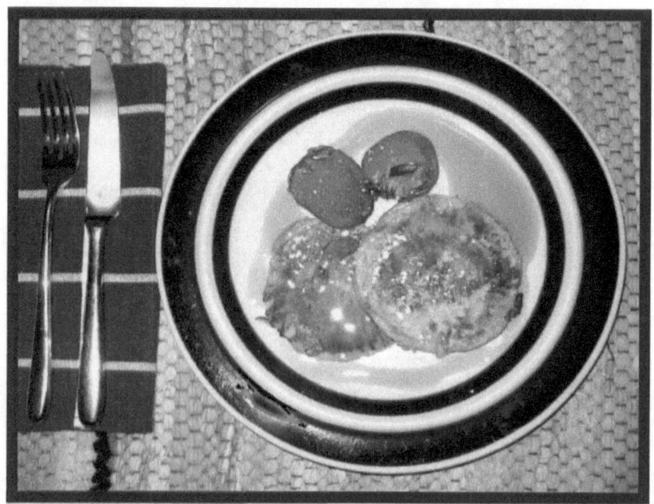

<u>Diet Tip of the Day:</u> **"Eat Slowly"** This is especially vital when you are trying to lose weight. If you are someone who eats fast, who finishes before everyone else at the table, you are not giving yourself a chance to feel full. While everyone else is still eating, you either sit there and pick, or you have seconds, taking in extra calories you could avoid if you would just slow down.

Day 3 Recipe

<u>Baked Herb-Crusted Cod</u>

4 cod fish fillets (4 to 5 ounces each)
2 tablespoons flour
2 tablespoons cornmeal
2 tablespoons minced fresh herbs
2 teaspoons lemon juice

Sprinkle cod with lemon juice. Mix flour, cornmeal and herbs and dust the cod with the cornmeal-herb mixture. Bake in oven at 375 ºF for 10 minutes. Add salt and black pepper to taste.
<u>Serves 4</u>. One serving is about 230 Calories (for cod only).

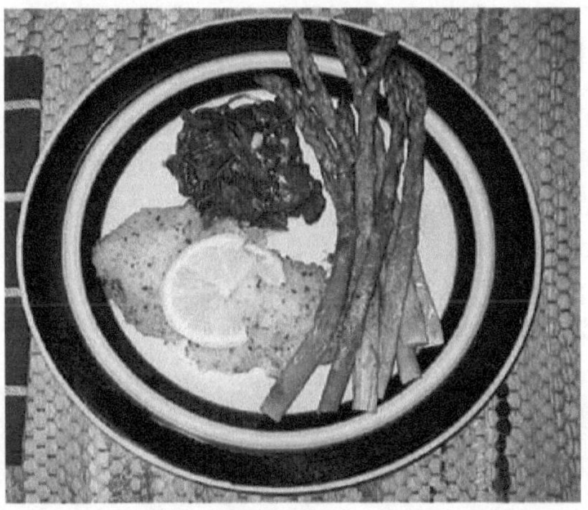

<u>**Diet Tip of the Day:**</u>. Successful weight loss and subsequent weight maintenance **requires knowledge, desire and discipline**. Avoid the latest fad diets. Instead, take the time to develop a true understanding of weight control and then change your eating and activity habits accordingly.

Day 4 Recipe

<u>Pasta and Veggies</u>

- ¾ pound penne pasta
- 2 cups broccoli florets
- 1 red bell pepper, sliced
- 1 carrot, cut to 1-inch sticks
- ½ cup frozen green peas & ½ cup frozen sweet corn
- 1 small onion, chopped
- 1 tablespoon minced garlic
- 3 tablespoons olive oil
- 1 teaspoon fresh basil, chopped

Cook penne pasta per package directions. Drain and place pasta in a bowl. Pre-cook the carrot and broccoli florets.

In a large heavy skillet, heat the olive oil and sauté onion and garlic until lightly golden. Add vegetables and sauté until the peppers are soft. Combine sautéed vegetables in the bowl with the pasta. Toss well. Garnish with chopped basil, season to taste, and top with freshly grated Parmesan cheese.

Serves 4. 460 Calories per serving

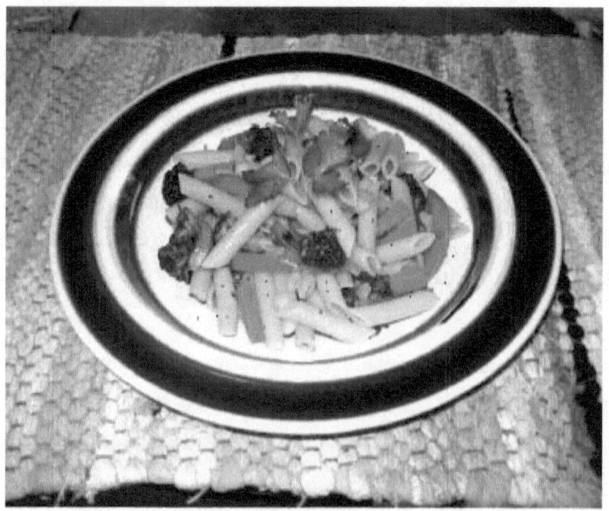

Photo taken before grated cheese was added.

Diet Tip of the Day: When possible, **select fresh and natural foods** and whole-grain products. Avoid chemical preservatives and additives, artificial and imitation foods, refined and processed foods, and foods that are comprised of "nutritionally-empty calories."

Day 5 Recipe
<u>Frozen-Fish Dinner</u>

No recipe today. No cooking today. It's your day off! To find a frozen fish dinner, please go to Appendix A (page 106) which lists approximately 150 frozen dinners manufactured by Healthy Choice, Lean Cuisine and Smart Ones.

Perusing the list, it is obvious that there are not many frozen fish dinners for sale at supermarkets. Note that if you do not use all of the **340 Calories allocated for this Day 5 meal**, use the excess calories anyway you wish. Splurge on extra dessert or save the calories for the next day and have a larger piece of pizza!

Please read the important **Frozen-Food Safety Warning** in Appendix B on page 113.

<u>**Diet Tip of the Day:**</u> **Buy a pedometer** and start walking. For the average person 2,100 steps amounts to walking about one mile. A Harvard study has shown that 8,000 to 10,000 step per day promote weight loss. And you're not obliged to walk continuously until you accrue all 10,000 steps. Rather, all steps throughout the day to wherever and whenever count toward your daily total. Because 10,000 steps a day may not be achievable by some people, particularly those who are elderly, sedentary, or who have chronic diseases, rather than insisting on a blanket 10,000 steps per day, your initial stepping goal should your baseline steps plus an increment of an additional 2,500 steps. (Your baseline being the number of steps you take in an average day.)

Day 6 Recipe

<u>Grandma's Pizza</u>

The following is a pizza recipe used by my Italian grandmother. She was from a small mountain village located between Rome and Naples.
Pizza dough: To save time use prepared dough, preferably whole wheat. Flour a large cutting board. <u>Divide one pound of prepared pizza dough into four parts</u>. Roll out each dough ball as thin as possible.
Tomato sauce: Sauté ½ small onion, chopped fine, in 1 tsp olive oil. Add two finely chopped garlic cloves, 1½ cups chopped plum tomatoes and ½ tsp chopped fresh oregano. Stir and cook about 5 minutes on a low flame.
Pizza preparation & cooking: On each pizza, spread evenly about ¼ cup of the tomato sauce. Add about ½ ounce of shredded part-skim mozzarella cheese, 1 tsp Parmesan cheese, 3 slices of a Portobello mushroom, some torn fresh basil, and drizzle with Evoo. Put pizzas on a pan and place in 475 °F oven for about 15 to 20 minutes, or until crust is crisp and cheese is just melting. (Freeze left over sauce for use on Day 13.)
<u>Serves 4</u>. Make four pizzas. Each pizza contains about 350 Calories.

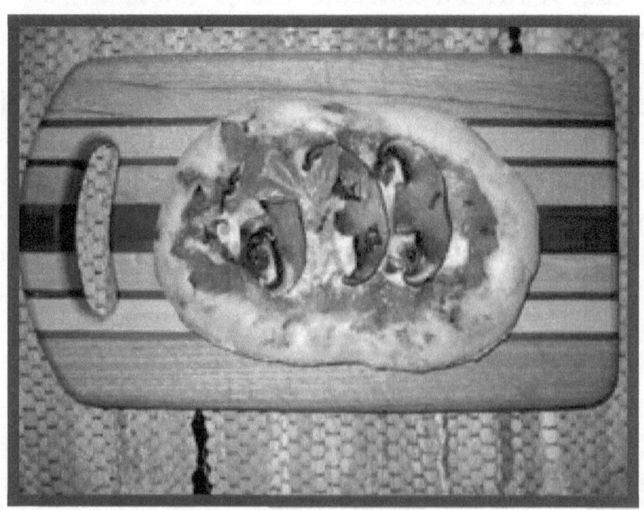

<u>Diet Tip of the Day:</u> For **life-long weight control** take a vigorous 30 to 60 minute walk everyday! That's right – everyday. Make exercise a nonflexible top priority part of your life. When it comes to exercise the key words are consistent, persistent, unyielding, dogged. Get the point?

Day 7 Recipe

<u>Chicken Dinner - Out</u>

No recipe today. No cooking today. Have a chicken dinner at your favorite restaurant, but make sure you choose a restaurant where you have a fighting chance to achieve your calorie goal. For 1200 Calorie meal plan, your goal for dinner is a **maximum of 580 Calories**. For 1500 Calorie meal plan, your goal for dinner is a **maximum of 630 Calories**. This includes appetizer, soup, main course, dessert and a glass of wine.

Tips for Eating Out: First, order simple, such as broiled chicken breast with steamed vegetables and brown rice. Tell the waiter you want no sauce, no gravy, nothing added. Then, knowing your calorie objective, and that chicken is about 50 Calories per ounce, most steamed vegetable servings average approximately 50 Calories per cup, and rice is about 100 Calories per ½ cup, decide how much to eat – and take the remainder home. If fresh fruit is not an option, pass on dessert and have the evening snack specified for that day in the diet.

In a restaurant, some nutritionists recommend you eat the low-calorie items on your plate first. Start with the salad, soup and veggies. By the time you get to the chicken and starches you will hopefully be full enough to be content with smaller portions of the higher-calorie choices.

Finally, some dieticians advise their dieting clients not to eat out. That's right. They believe eating at home is safer. But our thought is you have to eat out eventually so why not learn how while your resolve is high?

<u>Diet Tip of the Day:</u> When you're on a diet, eating in a restaurant can be a challenge, because most restaurant portions are huge, and can easily total more than 1,000 Calories. When eating in a restaurant decide how much to eat – and take the remainder home. A good general rule of thumb is to **eat half and bring the rest home**.

Day 8 Recipe

Baked Salmon with Salsa

This is a simple, straight-forward recipe. Again, the advantage of a simple recipe is there are no hidden calories.

   4 5 oz salmon fillets
   6 Tbsp bottled tomato-pepper salsa

Brown salmon fillets in non-stick pan and place in baking dish. Put fillets in an oven preheated to 350 ºF for about 10 minutes. Plate the salmon. Stir prepared tomato-pepper salsa and spoon it over the salmon.
Serves 4. One salmon fillet is about 215 Calories.

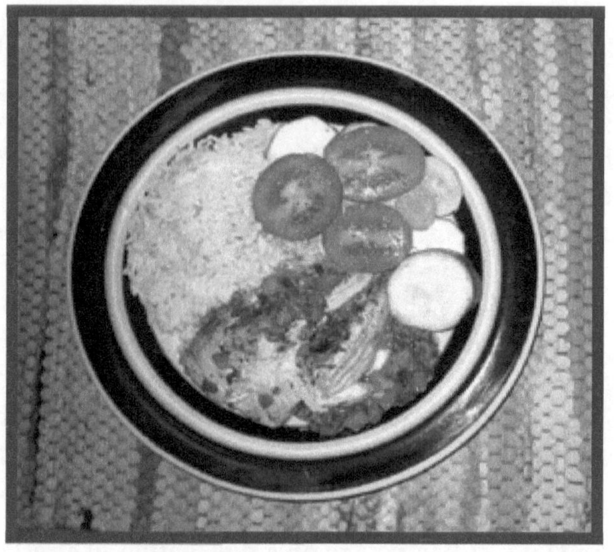

Diet Tip of the Day: **Have soup more often.** Most non-cream-based soups are filling and low-calorie.

Day 9 Recipe

<u>Veggie Burger</u>

Vegetable-based burgers can be purchased at your local supermarket. The patty of a veggie burger can be made from vegetables, soy, nuts, mushrooms, textured vegetable protein, dairy, or a combination of these foods.

Two popular veggie burgers are the Boca Burger and Gardenburger. The Boca Burger is made chiefly from soy protein and wheat gluten. (Boca Burger patties are 2.5 oz each and range from 60 to 90 Calories.) The original Gardenburger is made from mushrooms, onions, brown rice, rolled oats, cheese, and spices. (Gardenburger patties are 2.5 oz each and about 100 Calories.)

To prepare, follow package directions. The version shown below has an added slice of low-fat cheddar cheese. The lettuce, tomato and ketchup shown actually add very few extra calories.

The veggie burger patty plus low-fat cheese amounts to approximately 150 Calories. Add a seeded roll and the total rises to 290 Calories.

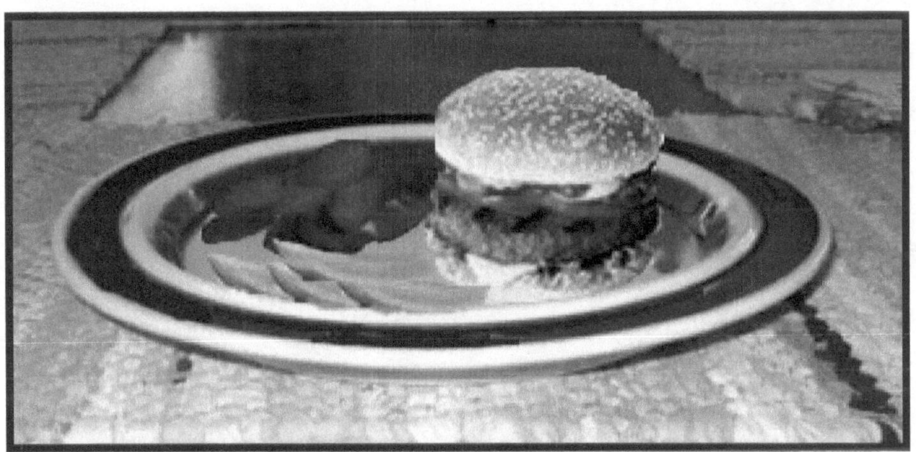

<u>Diet Tip of the Day:</u> **Drink lots of water** – about 8 glasses per day. Add a slice of lemon to make it more interesting. Often, when you think you're hungry, you are just thirsty. So, next time you head for a snack, drink some water first and see if that does it for you.

Day 10 Recipe

<u>Wild Blueberry Pancakes</u>

This recipe makes a relatively low calorie, wholesome batch of delicious wild blueberry-whole wheat-buttermilk pancakes.

  1 cup whole-wheat flour
  1 cup buttermilk
  1 egg
  1 Tbsp vegetable oil
  1 tsp baking powder
  ½ tsp baking soda

Stir ingredients until blended. Add ¾ cup blueberries and gently stir. Using medium heat, preheat a non-stick skillet coated with cooking spray (see page 9). Pour slightly less than ¼ cup of batter onto skillet per pancake. Cook slowly until bubbles break on surface of pancake. Turn and cook until other side is lightly browned. Makes 8 pancakes. Pictured below are wild-blueberry pancakes with two slices of turkey bacon.

<u>Serves 4</u>. Each pancake is about 95 Calories

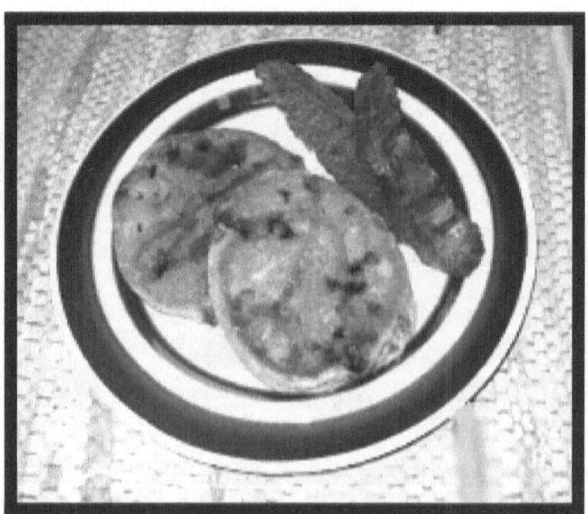

<u>Diet Tip of the Day:</u> A peanut butter sandwich on whole wheat bread with a glass of skim milk and an apple makes a nutritious, reasonably low-calorie lunch.

Day 11 Recipe

Artichoke-Bean Salad

1 can (19 oz) white kidney beans
10 artichoke hearts, quartered
⅓ cup chopped oregano
⅓ cup chopped parsley
3 cloves garlic, chopped
1 lemon, juiced

Combine ingredients in medium-size bowl. Stir in ¼ cup Evoo. Salt and black pepper to taste.

Serves 6. Artichoke-bean salad has approximately 190 Calories per serving.

Pictured on the plate below are two grilled chicken sausage links with salsa, steamed green beans and the artichoke-bean salad. Incidentally, this artichoke-bean combination over mixed salad greens served with a whole-grain bread makes a delicious, nutritious and reasonable low-calorie main course.

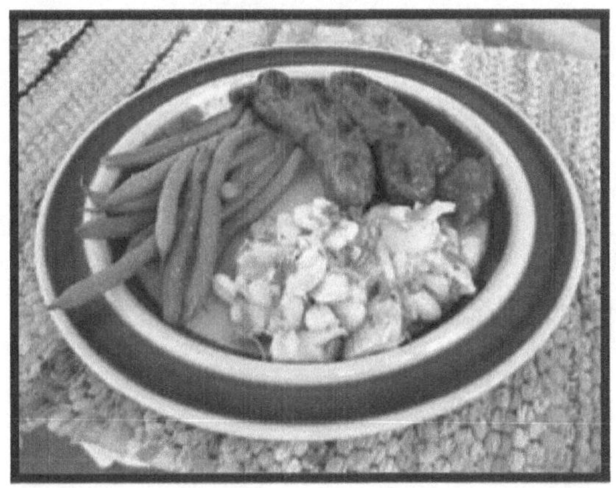

Diet Tip of the Day: Have a small meal before you go to a party. A hardboiled egg, an apple, and a thirst quencher (like water, tea, seltzer, or diet soda) will take the edge off your appetite and make it easier to resist the high-calorie goodies.

Day 12 Recipe

<u>Fish Dinner - Out</u>

No recipe today. No cooking today. Have a fish dinner at your favorite restaurant, but make sure you choose a restaurant where you have a good chance to achieve your calorie goal. For Day 12, your **goal for dinner is a maximum of 595 Calories**. This includes appetizer, soup, main course, dessert and a glass of wine.

Tips for Eating Out: The following is almost an exact repeat of advice given for Day 7. First, order simple, such as broiled fish with steamed vegetables and brown rice. Tell the waiter you want no sauce, no gravy, nothing added. Then, knowing your calorie objective, and that fish is about 50 Calories per ounce, most steamed vegetable servings average approximately 50 Calories per cup, and rice is about 100 Calories per ½ cup, decide how much to eat – and take the remainder home. If fresh fruit is not an option, pass on dessert and have the evening snack specified for that day in the diet.

In a restaurant, I recommend you eat the low-calorie items on your plate first. Start with the salad, soup and veggies. By the time you get to the fish and starches you will hopefully be full enough to be content with smaller portions of the higher-calorie choices.

<u>Diet Tip of the Day:</u> Phytonutrients are found in plant foods such as fruits, vegetables, whole grains, dried beans, nuts and seeds. Unlike protein, fat, vitamins and minerals, phytonutrients are not necessary for life, but evidence is growing that phytonutrients have many beneficial qualities.

Day 13 Recipe

<u>Pasta with Marinara Sauce</u>

Prepare the sauce as you did for the Day 6 pizza. But because the pizza sauce is a bit too thick, add ¼ cup of pasta liquid to thin it. (The spiral pasta shape shown below is called Fusilli, and is a favorite because all the ridges really hold the sauce.)

    ½ pound <u>whole-wheat</u> pasta

    ¼ tsp salt

Prepare the marinara tomato sauce as per Day 6 sauce but dilute it with ¼ cup of pasta liquid. Bring 2 quarts of lightly salted water to a boil. Add pasta and stir occasionally (to keep pasta from sticking to the bottom of the pot). Keep water boiling and cook until pasta are "al dente." (Cooking time is approximately 9 minutes.) Drain pasta, add marinara sauce and serve hot.

<u>Serves 4</u>. One serving is about 225 Calories.

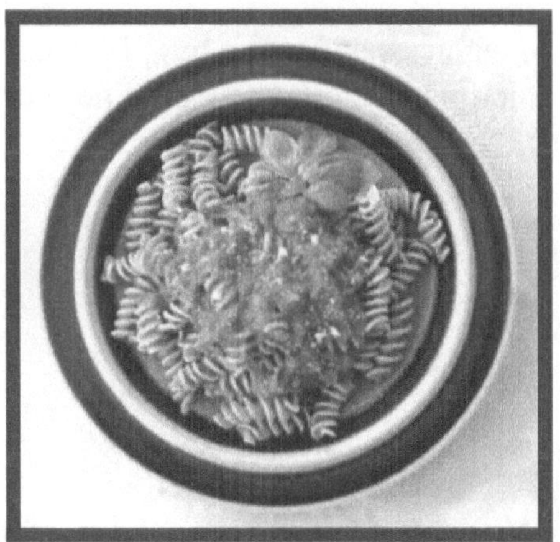

<u>Diet Tip of the Day:</u> **Beware of alcoholic beverages**. Beer has about 13 Calories per ounce, wine 25 Calories per ounce and whiskey 71 Calories per ounce.

Day 14 Recipe

<u>"Oatena" Cereal Mix</u>

Mixing nutritious cereals, hot or cold, is a good way to add variety as well as nutrition to a meal. This recipe features a mix of two whole grain cereals: Oatmeal and Wheatena.

    ⅓ cup Oatmeal
    ¼ cup (4 Tbsp) Wheatena
    ¾ cup water
    ½ cup skim milk
    ¼ cup blueberries
    10 raisins

Add Oatmeal, Wheatena, raisins and a dash of salt to a microwave-safe cereal bowl. Next add water and stir. Place bowl in microwave, on high power for about 1½ minutes, or until desired consistency is reached. The result is "Oatena," a mix of oatmeal and Wheatena, shown (half eaten) below.

Add skim milk and blueberries and serve hot. Because of the natural sugar in blueberries and raisins, adding sugar is not necessary.

<u>Serves 1</u>. About 310 Calories per serving

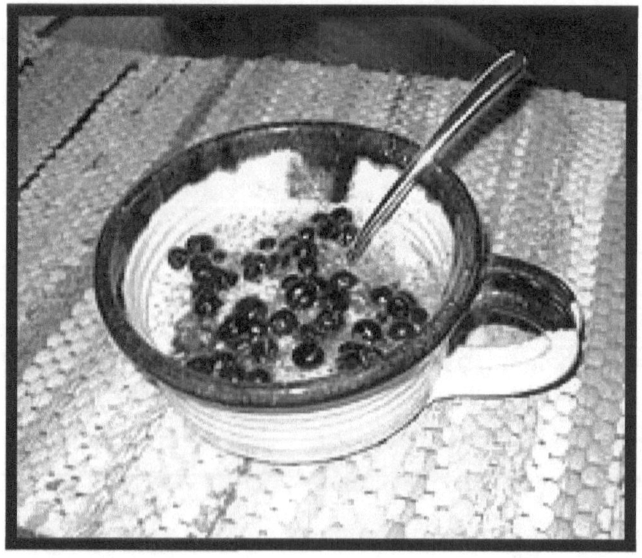

<u>Diet Tip of the Day:</u> Hot or cold cereal topped with fruit, and fat-free milk makes a nutritious, relatively low-calorie meal anytime.

Day 15 Recipe

<u>Tuna & Bean Salad</u>

1 tuna steak, about 2 inches thick (14 ounces)
2 tablespoons extra-virgin olive oil
1 tablespoon lemon juice
1 garlic clove, crushed
1 tablespoon Dijon mustard
1 15-ounce can cannellini beans, drained
1 small red onion, thinly sliced
2 red peppers, seeded and thinly sliced
½ cucumber, halved lengthwise and thinly sliced
6 cups watercress

Heat a ridged grill pan coated with cooking spray (see page 9) over medium-high heat. Season tuna steak on both sides with coarsely ground black pepper. Cook the tuna 4 minutes on each side - the outside should be browned and the center light pink. Be careful not to overcook. Remove from the pan and set aside.

Mix together the oil, lemon juice, garlic, and mustard in a salad bowl. Season with salt and pepper to taste. Add the cannellini beans, onion, peppers, cucumber and watercress. Toss gently to mix. Cut tuna into ½-inch thick slices. Arrange on top of salad and serve with lemon wedges. **<u>Serves 4</u>**. 355 Calories per serving

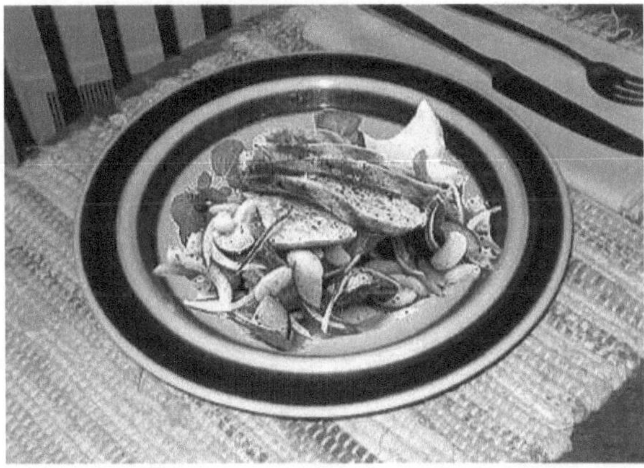

<u>**Diet Tip of the Day:**</u> In the United States, for a food to be labeled "**whole grain**" it must contain more than 51 percent whole grain by weight.

Day 16 Recipe

<u>Baked Red Snapper</u>

 4 red snapper fillets – 4 oz each (salmon may be substituted)
 ½ cup white wine
 ½ cup non-fat yogurt mixed with half as much mustard
 ½ pound green beans
 20 cherry tomatoes
 4 tsp olive oil
 1 cup wild rice, brown rice and wheat berry mix

Prepare rice mix per package directions.

Brown fillets in non-stick pan. Place fillets skin side down in baking dish coated with non-stick spray (see page 9). Add white wine and cook in oven preheated to 350 ºF for about 15 minutes. Spoon pan juices over fillets. Salt and pepper to taste.

Place green beans in skillet. Add ¼-inch of water and cook over medium heat until water boils off. Add cherry tomatoes and olive oil. Stir well and sauté for a few minutes. Season with fresh rosemary and oregano. Salt and pepper to taste.

Plate red snapper fillet and spoon over yogurt-mustard sauce. Add green beans & tomato mix and the wild rice. Serve hot.

<u>Serves 4</u>. One plate consisting of one snapper fillet (215 Calories) with green beans & tomato mix (75 Calories) and wild rice (160 Calories) totals 450 Calories.

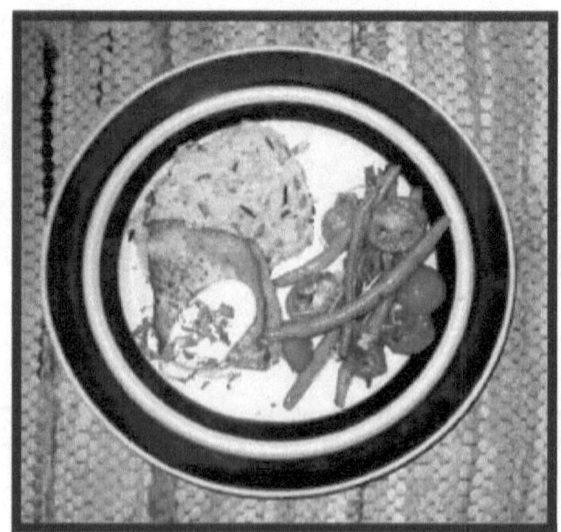

<u>Diet Tip of the Day:</u> **Don't have sweets in your house**. This makes them easier to resist. Out of sight, out of mind!

Day 17 Recipe

Cajun Chicken Salad

This is a perfect after-work, quick, nutritious and delicious dinner.

  4 boneless and skinless chicken breasts (about 5 oz each)
  1 bottle Cajun spices
  8 ounces mixed salad greens
  20 cherry tomatoes
  12 pitted black olives

Brush chicken breasts lightly with olive oil. Roll breasts in Cajun spices.
Brown breasts on non-stick oven-proof skillet. After breasts are brown,
put skillet in 350 °F oven for approximately 15 minutes, or until done. Cut
breasts into ½-inch slices. (When the breasts are done, the meat should be
moist and white with no sign of pink.) Serve hot or keep in an oven or
warmer at 200 °F until ready to plate.

Place chicken slices over a bed of mixed salad greens. Add tomatoes,
olives and 2 Tbsp of your favorite low-calorie salad dressing.

Serves 4. 330 Calories per serving.

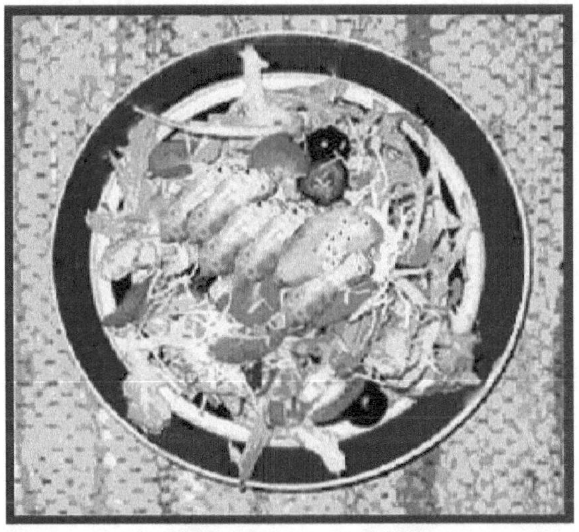

Diet Tip of the Day: Know that **fat-free isn't always your best bet**.
Very often sugar is substituted for fat and the calorie total remains the
same. Low fat does not necessarily mean low calorie! Rather, look for
low-calorie or reduced-calorie products.

Day 18 Recipe

<u>Grilled Swordfish</u>

1¼ pounds swordfish
1 bottle citrus-herb marinade
24 cherry tomatoes
4 medium potatoes
2 cups fresh spinach
1 tsp rosemary & juice of ¼ lemon
2 tsp extra virgin olive oil (Evoo)

Steam spinach with garlic and drizzle with Evoo. Cut up potatoes and place sprinkle with lemon juice, add rosemary, salt and black pepper. Place on grill for about 10 minutes, turning occasionally.

Toss cherry tomatoes in small amount Evoo. Add fresh oregano, salt and black pepper. Place on heavy-duty aluminum foil, seal and grill for about 3 minutes.

Marinade swordfish in citrus-herb vinaigrette. Grill on hot fire for about 5 minutes on one side and 3 minutes on the other, or until done as desired.

Serves 4. One plate consisting of grilled swordfish (250 Calories) with grilled potatoes (100 Calories) and cherry tomatoes (45 Calories) and steamed spinach (50 Calories) totals 445 Calories.

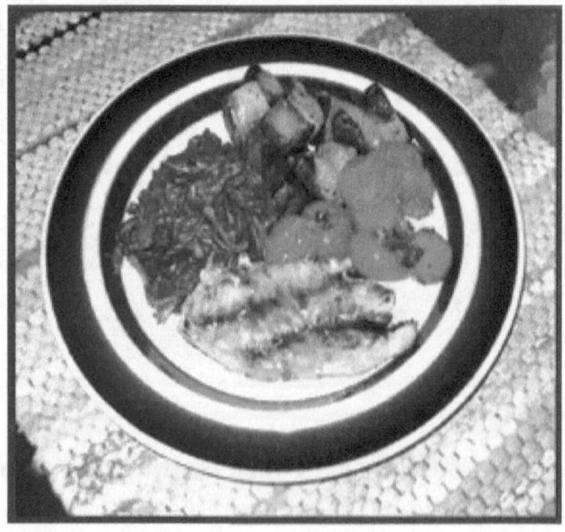

<u>Diet Tip of the Day:</u> Don't be in a hurry to lose weight. Slow weight loss is healthier, is more likely to be permanent, and is easier to sustain over the long haul.

Day 19 Recipe

<u>Italian Food - Out</u>

No recipe today. No cooking today. Have dinner at your favorite Italian restaurant, but make sure you choose a restaurant where you have a reasonable chance to achieve your calorie goal. For today, **your goal for dinner is a maximum of 640 Calories**. This includes any appetizer, soup, main course and a 4 oz glass of red wine.

Tips for Eating Italian: You can consume a lot of calories in an Italian restaurant – if you order carelessly. For example a typical portion is often loaded with about 1000 Calories, then add another 100 Calories for a glass of wine.

First rule, order simple. Look for a dish with lots of vegetables, some fish or chicken. Then, knowing your 640 Calorie objective, and that chicken and fish are about 50 Calories per ounce, most steamed vegetable servings average approximately 50 Calories per cup, and pasta is about 200 Calories per cup, decide how much of the meal you can eat – and take the remainder home. Pass on dessert and have the evening snack specified for that day in the diet. Also see **Eating Out** (page 10) for more guidance.

<u>**Diet Tip of the Day:**</u>   Another dilemma for dieters is **judging portion size**. It makes no sense to worry about whether to apportion 70 or 80 Calories per ounce for a cut of lean meat if you have no idea whether the portion you are planning to eat weighs four or ten ounces. To be successful, you must learn to estimate portion sizes with reasonable accuracy.

Day 20 Recipe

<u>Quick Pasta alla Puttanesca</u>

This famous pasta dish originated in Naples. Puttanesca means "ladies of the night." The exact origin of the name is unclear, but one thing is clear: It's delicious! Here is one of many recipe versions.

  ½ pound spaghetti (whole wheat preferred)
  20 black pitted olives
  1 can (14½ oz) diced tomatoes
  ½ can (4 oz) tomato sauce
  2 Tbsp Evoo
  3 cloves of garlic, chopped and 1Tbsp dried minced onion
  ½ tsp crushed red pepper flakes
  1 Tbsp capers drained and rinsed
  ¼ cup currants

Cook spaghetti according to package directions. Drain and return spaghetti to pot; add a teaspoon Evoo and toss to coat.

Heat 2 tablespoons olive oil in large skillet over medium-high heat. Add red pepper flakes; cook and stir 1 to 2 minutes or until sizzling. Add onion and garlic; cook and stir 1 minute. Finally, add tomatoes with juice, tomato sauce, olives, currants and capers. Cook over medium-high heat, stirring frequently, until sauce is heated through.

<u>Serves 4</u>. About 345 Calories per serving

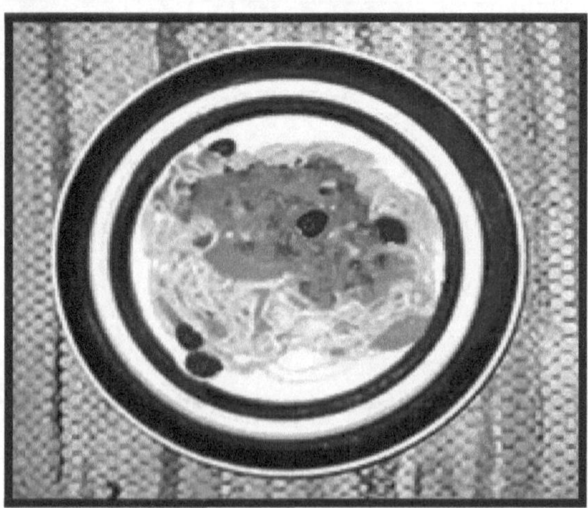

<u>Diet Tip of the Day:</u> Dilute juices, such as apple juice, orange, etc. with water. This cuts the flavor slightly but really reduces calorie content.

Day 21 Recipe

<u>Frozen-Meat Dinner</u>

No recipe today. No cooking today. It's your day off! To find a frozen meat dinner entrée please go to Appendix A (page 106) which lists approximately 150 frozen dinners manufactured by Healthy Choice, Lean Cuisine and Smart Ones.

Note that if you do not use all of the **300 Calories allocated for the Day 21 frozen dinner**, use the excess calories anyway you wish. Splurge on extra dessert or save the calories for another day.

Please read the important **Frozen-Food Safety Warning** in Appendix B on page 113.

<u>**Diet Tip of the Day:**</u> A good understanding of nutrition is not only vital for good health but also will help you control your weight over the long term. For example, did you know that foods that are an "excellent source" of a particular nutrient provide 20% or more of the Recommended Daily Value. Whereas, foods that are a "good source" of a nutrient provide between 10 and 20% of the Recommended Daily Value.

Day 22 Recipe

<u>Shrimp & Spinach Salad</u>

2 pounds shrimp in shell
½ pound small green beans, trimmed
½ pound baby spinach leaves
2 Tbsp lemon juice
¼ cup Evoo
2 tsp minced fresh dill
1 Tbsp minced green onion

To make vinaigrette, combine lemon juice, olive oil, dill, salt and pepper to taste and whisk until blended. Stir in minced onion and set aside.

Peel, de-vein and butterfly shrimp. Place shrimp in a bowl and add water to cover. Add 1 teaspoon of salt, and let stand for 10 minutes. Drain, rinse, drain again, and dry. Arrange shrimp in broiling pan without a rack. Brush shrimp with a little vinaigrette and place under preheated broiler, about 3 inches from heat. Broil about 3 to 4 minutes, turning shrimp once, or until both sides turn pink.

Remove shrimp from broiler and add remaining vinaigrette and green beans to the broiling pan. Stir to coat shrimp and beans with vinaigrette. Pour warm vinaigrette over spinach and toss quickly. Plate the spinach and arrange shrimp and green beans on top.

<u>Serves 4</u>. 310 Calories per serving.

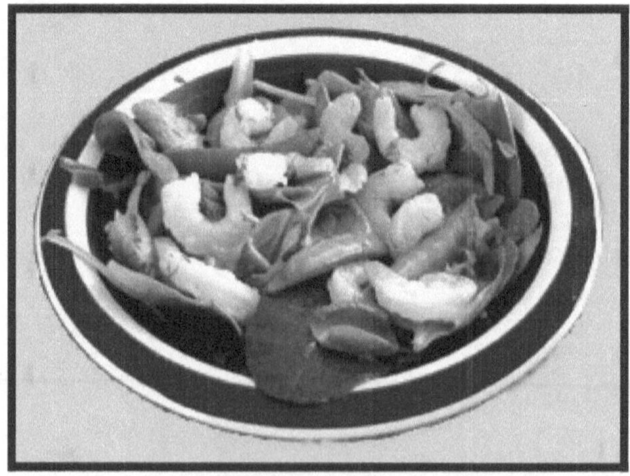

<u>Diet Tip of the Day:</u> After company leaves, have them take some of the leftover food (particularly the dessert) with them – or take the leftovers to work the next day.

Day 23 Recipe

<u>Beans & Greens Salad</u>

⅓ cup chopped oregano
⅓ cup chopped parsley
3 cloves garlic, chopped
1 lemon, juiced
Prepare salad dressing by combining above ingredients and stirring in ¼
cup Evoo. Salt and pepper to taste.
½ pound mesclun mix
¼ pound green beans
1 19 oz can garbanzo beans (chickpeas)
Arrange mesclun mix, garbanzo beans and green beans on a large platter.
Drizzle salad dressing over beans and greens.
<u>Serves 4</u>. Approximately 260 Calories per serving.

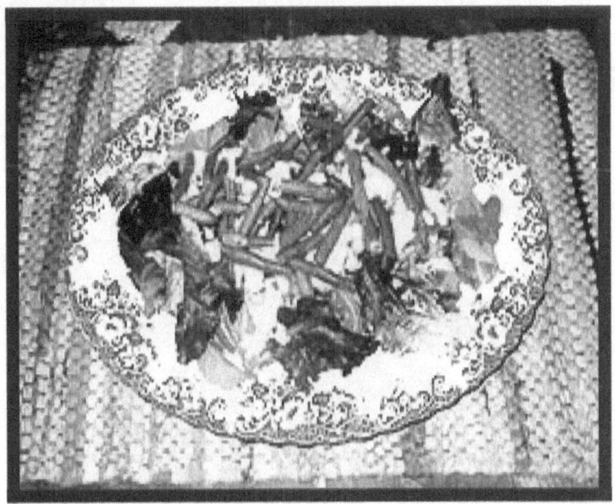

<u>Diet Tip of the Day:</u> Beans are a wonderful food but they are an
incomplete protein. If however beans are eaten with a whole-grain bread,
the combination forms a complete protein – just as complete and nutritious
as meat, poultry, or fish.

Day 24 Recipe

<u>Four-Bean Plus Salad</u>

Note that the total caloric value of the salad will change very little, if the proportions of the bean varieties and corn are varied – according to taste.

  ½ cup canned red kidney beans, drained and rinsed
  ½ cup canned black beans, drained and rinsed
  ½ cup canned chick peas, drained and rinsed
  ½ cup canned cannelloni beans, drained and rinsed
  ½ cup canned corn, drained
  1 small red pepper, chopped
  1 small green pepper, chopped
  2 Tbsp Evoo
  2 Tbsp lemon juice

In a large bowl mix red kidney beans, black beans, chick peas, cannelloni beans, corn and chopped red and green peppers. Stir in Evoo and lemon juice and plate.

<u>**Serves about 6**</u>. One serving is ½ cup – with about 135 Calories per serving

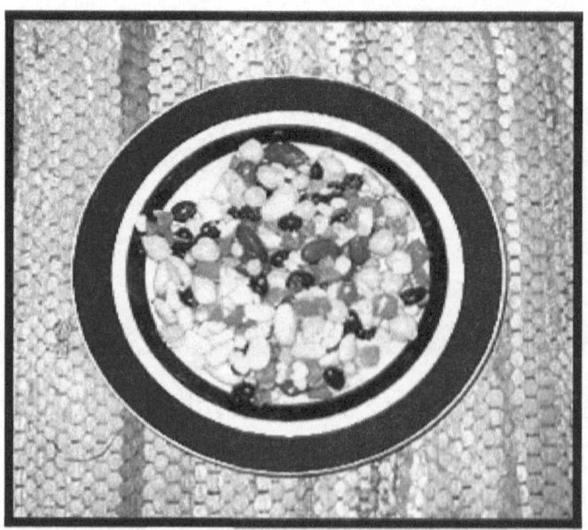

<u>**Diet Tip of the Day:**</u> Vigorous exercise doesn't necessarily stimulate you to overeat. Just the opposite. In many cases, exercise actually helps curb your appetite – immediately following a workout.

Day 25 Recipe

<u>Pan-Broiled Hanger Steak</u>

1¼ pounds hanger steak, well trimmed of fat
¼ cup lime juice
8 small new potatoes, peeled and halved
12 cherry tomatoes, cut in half

Season both sides of steak with salt and pepper and place in sealable plastic bag with lime juice. Refrigerate for about one hour.
Boil potatoes about 10 minutes. Rinse in cold water. Sauté potatoes in small amount of vegetable oil over medium-high heat until brown.
Sauté cherry tomatoes in small amount of olive oil over medium-high heat until skin begins to crack. Season with chopped fresh basil.
Heat a skillet over medium-high heat. Sear hanger steak on one side for about 5 minutes. Turn over and sear other side approximately 5 minutes (for medium done). Pour off any fat that may have accumulated. Carve into ½-inch slices.
<u>Serves 4.</u> About 320 Calories per serving (for the hanger steak only)

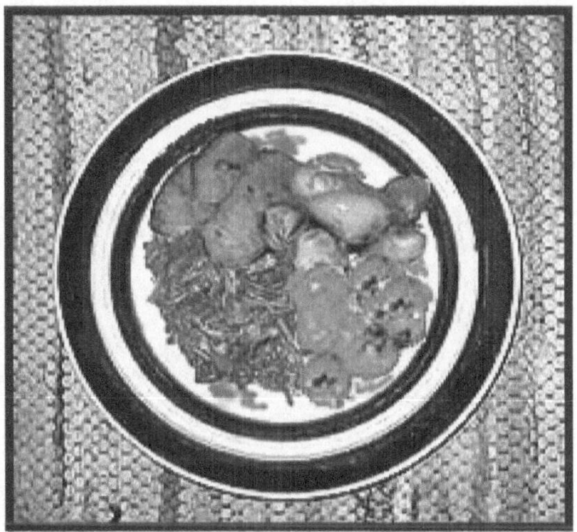

<u>Diet Tip of the Day:</u> If you find yourself at a party, don't stand near the food! Be aware of the temptation. Make the effort, and you'll find you eat less.

Day 26 Recipe

<u>Grilled Scallops and Polenta</u>

   1 pound sea scallops
   ¾ cup polenta cornmeal
   ¾ cup skim milk
   1 medium Portobello mushroom
   ½ pound green beans
   ¼ cup chopped red onion
   16 asparagus spear
   1 tsp Evoo

Bring 1½ cups of water and skim milk to rapid boil. Add salt to taste and slowly add polenta while stirring. Reduce heat. Continue stirring until desired consistency is reached. Pour polenta into lightly greased pan. After polenta has cooled cover and refrigerate. Cut chilled polenta into 4 pieces. Grill on medium-hot fire – about two minutes on each side. Brush Portobello mushroom and asparagus spear with Evoo and place on grill for about 3 minutes on each side.

Grill scallops on medium-hot fire. Turn after two minutes or when first side turns opaque. Grill until second side turns opaque – about another 2 minutes. Don't overcook but test a scallop by cutting to make sure it's cooked through. Salt and pepper to taste.

<u>Serves 4</u>. The food on the plate pictured below totals 380 Calories.

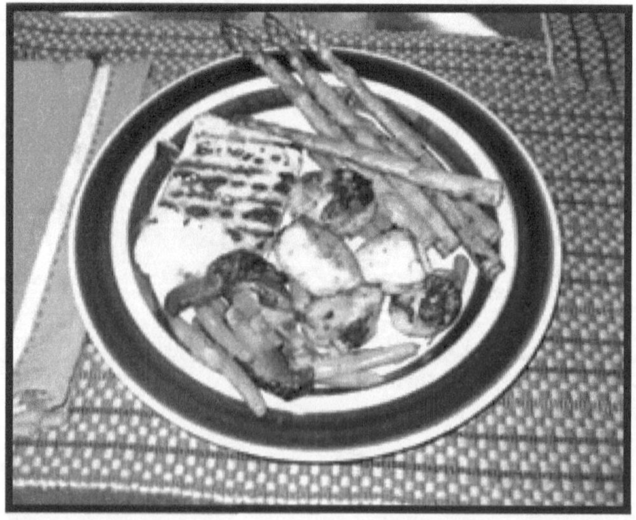

<u>Diet Tip of the Day:</u> To have better control of what you eat **bring your lunch to work**.

Day 27 Recipe
<u>Fettuccine in Summer Sauce</u>

This sauce is often served in the summer because it's lighter than what is usually dished up with pasta. But despite its name the sauce is wonderful year round.

  ½ pound fettuccine
  8 ounces fresh asparagus, trimmed & cut into 2" pieces
  20 cherry tomatoes, halved
  2 Tbsp plus 1 tsp Evoo
  2 cloves of garlic, chopped
  ½ small onion, diced

Cook fettuccine according to package directions. Drain and return pasta to pot; add a teaspoon Evoo and toss to coat. Meanwhile steam asparagus and drain.

In large skillet over medium-high heat, sauté cherry tomatoes in 2 Tbsp olive oil until skin begins to crack. Add onion and cook until translucent. Stir in garlic . Thin sauce with pasta liquid to desired consistency. Toss cooked pasta and asparagus into sauce and serve immediately.

<u>Serves 4</u>. About 290 Calories per serving

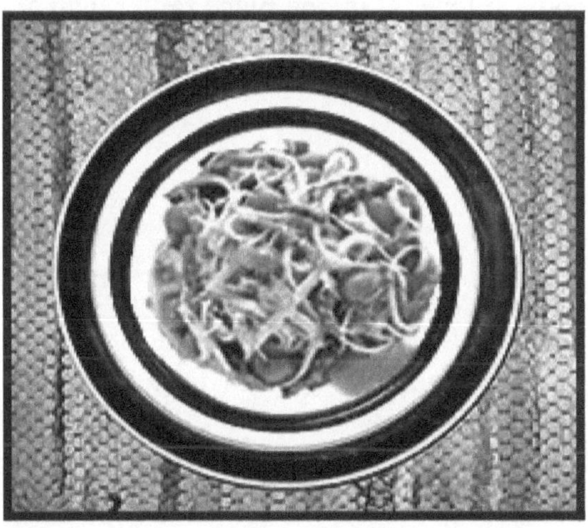

<u>Diet Tip of the Day:</u> A major weight-loss fallacy is that you can get rid of abdominal fat by working your abdominal muscles. This is based on the incorrect belief that fat is eliminated from a particular part of your body if you engage the muscles underneath that layer of fat. No such luck.

Day 28 Recipe

<u>**Frozen Chicken Meal**</u>

No recipe today. No cooking today. It's your day off! To find a frozen chicken dinner entrée please go to Appendix A (page 106) which lists approximately 150 frozen dinners manufactured by Healthy Choice, Lean Cuisine and Smart Ones.

Note that if you do not use all of the **300 Calories allocated for the Day 14 and 28 frozen dinner**, use the excess calories anyway you wish. Splurge on extra dessert or save the calories for another day.

Please read the important **Frozen-Food Safety Warning** in Appendix B on page 113.

<u>**Diet Tip of the Day:**</u>   The **general weight-change rule is "last on first off."** Assume as you gained weight, the first place you noticed it was on your thighs, next your buttocks, then your face. As you lose weight, it generally will come off in the reverse order, first from your face, then your rear and finally your thighs. And there is not much you can do about that. The truth is there is no food, no exercise, no magic belt, and no pill that will cause your body to lose fat in one place rather than another.

Day 29 Recipe

<u>Barbequed Shrimp</u>

1½ pounds large shrimp
3 Tbsp bottled barbeque sauce
4 medium ears of corn

Pour barbeque sauce into shallow bowl. Toss shrimp in barbeque sauce to coat. Place shrimp on medium-hot grill. Turn shrimp after about two minutes or when shrimp turn pink. Grill until second side turns pink – approximately another 2 minutes. Don't overcook but test a shrimp by cutting to make sure it is cooked through. Salt and pepper to taste. Serve hot or at room temperature.

Serves 4. About 160 Calories per serving (shrimp only).

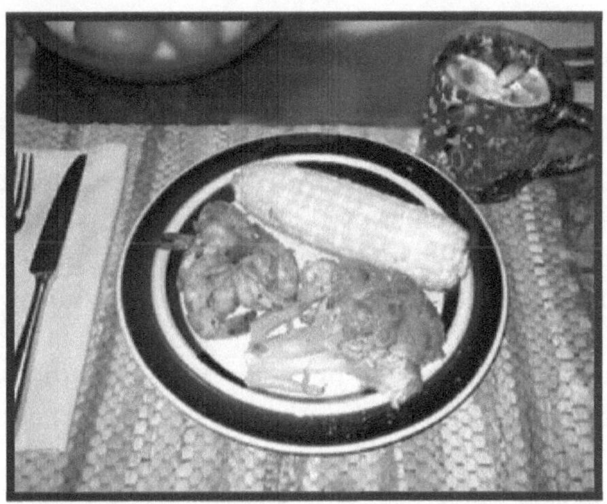

<u>Diet Tip of the Day:</u> A very important weight-profile parameter is your waist-to-hip ratio. Health risks for heart attack and stroke increase considerably for men with a ratio above 1.0 and for women with a ratio above 0.8. To calculate your ratio, measure your waist size (at its narrowest circumference) and divide it by your hip size (at the widest wedge).

Day 30 Recipe

<u>Pasta e Fagioli</u>

This is one variation of a traditional, nutritious peasant dish served in Italy.

    14.5-oz can whole tomatoes with juice, crushed
    14.5-oz can cannellini beans, drained
    1   cup of any tube-shaped pasta
    2   tablespoon olive oil
    1   medium onion, diced
    2   cloves garlic, minced
    1   stalk celery, finely chopped
    3   cups chicken stock
    2   cups fresh baby spinach or escarole
    1   tsp dried basil
    ½   teaspoon dried oregano
    2   Tbsp fresh parsley, chopped

Heat olive oil, onion and celery in large saucepan over medium heat. Sauté until onions are golden brown. Add garlic and stir constantly for one minute. Pour in tomatoes and their juices and bring to a boil. Add beans and chicken stock and return to a boil. Stir in spinach (or escarole) and seasonings. Simmer for about 5 minutes. Add pasta and cook about 15 minutes or until pasta is tender but firm. If needed, thin soup with hot water. Ladle into soup bowls. Garnish with grated Parmesan cheese. Salt and pepper to taste.

Serves 4. About 300 Calories per serving.

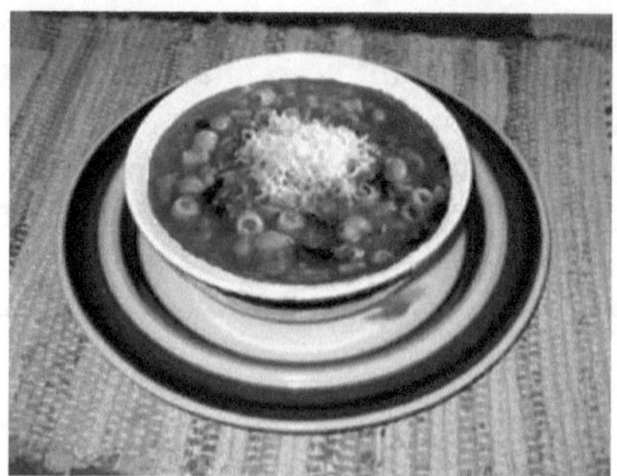

<u>Diet Tip of the Day</u>: Pasta alone is an incomplete protein. But when combined with beans, a complete protein results – that is a protein that contains all eight essential amino acids. The dish is every bit as nutritious as meat, fish or poultry.

APPENDIX A
Frozen Entrées

Appendix A lists three popular brands of frozen entrées: Healthy Choice, Lean Cuisine and Smart Ones. The listing is further divided by entrée type: Poultry entrées, Meat entrées, Seafood entrées, Pasta entrées, Pizza and Other entrées. The entire table is arranged from the lowest to highest in calories. Note that the listed frozen entrées were available in most super markets as of 08/23/2020.

Entrée Type	Name	Brand	Calories
Poultry	Tomato Basil Chicken & Spinach	Smart Ones	160
Poultry	Chicken Santa Fe	Smart Ones	160
Meat	Asian Style Beef & Broccoli	Smart Ones	160
Meat	Steak Portobella	Lean Cuisine	160
Seafood	Shrimp Alfredo	Lean Cuisine	160
Poultry	Herb Roasted Chicken	Lean Cuisine	170
Poultry	Chipotle Lime Chicken	Smart Ones	170
Poultry	Grilled Chicken Marsala	Healthy Choice	180
Poultry	Creamy Basil Chicken & Broccoli	Smart Ones	180
Poultry	Pomegranate Chicken	Lean Cuisine	180
Meat	Sweet Siracha Braised Beef	Lean Cuisine	180
Meat	Beef Merlot	Healthy Choice	180
Meat	Homestyle Beef Pot Roast	Smart Ones	180
Poultry	Roasted Turkey & Vegetables	Lean Cuisine	190
Poultry	Chicken & Broccoli Alfredo	Healthy Choice	190
Poultry	Chicken & Vegetable Stir Fry	Healthy Choice	190
Other	Broccoli & Cheddar Roast Potato	Smart Ones	190
Poultry	Home Style Chicken & Potatoes	Healthy Choice	200
Poultry	Crustless Chicken Pot Pie	Smart Ones	200
Poultry	Cheddar Bacon Chicken	Lean Cuisine	200
Pasta	Pasta Primavera	Smart Ones	200
Poultry	Slow Roasted Turkey Breast	Smart Ones	210

Poultry	Lemon Herb Chicken Piccata	Smart Ones	210
Poultry	Honey Balsamic Chicken	Healthy Choice	210
Pasta	Ravioli Florentine	Smart Ones	210
Poultry	Cajun Style Chicken & Shrimp	Healthy Choice	220
Poultry	Chicken Margherita	Smart Ones	220
Meat	Roast Beef & Mashed Potatoes	Smart Ones	220
Pasta	Creamy Pasta Romano	Smart Ones	220
Meat	Roast Beef & Mashed Potatoes	Smart Ones	220
Meat	Meat Loaf with Mashed Potatoes	Lean Cuisine	230
Meat	Pulled Pork & Black Beans	Smart Ones	230
Seafood	Shrimp & Angel Hair Pasta	Lean Cuisine	230
Pasta	Cheese Ravioli Mushroom Sauce	Smart Ones	230
Poultry	Chicken Carbonara	Lean Cuisine	240
Poultry	Creamy Basil Chick & Tortenllini	Lean Cuisine	240
Poultry	Glazed Chicken	Lean Cuisine	240
Poultry	Honey Glazed Turkey & Potatoes	Healthy Choice	240
Pasta	Spicy Penne Arrabbiata	Lean Cuisine	240
Pasta	Cheese Ravioli	Lean Cuisine	250
Pasta	Vermont Cheddar Mac & Cheese	Lean Cuisine	250
Pasta	Fettuccini Alfredo	Smart Ones	250
Pasta	Lasagna Bake with Meat Sauce	Smart Ones	250
Poultry	Fiesta Grilled Chicken	Lean Cuisine	250
Poultry	Baked Chicken	Lean Cuisine	250
Pasta	Chicken Linguini Red Pepper	Healthy Choice	250
Poultry	Golden Roasted Turkey Breast	Healthy Choice	250
Poultry	Chicken Mesquite	Smart Ones	250
Poultry	Chicken Oriental	Smart Ones	250
Poultry	Orange Sesame Chicken	Smart Ones	250
Poultry	Teriyaki Chicken & Vegetables	Smart Ones	250
Seafood	Tuna Noodle Casserole	Smart Ones	250

Category	Meal	Brand	Calories
Poultry	Grilled Chicken Primavera	Lean Cuisine	260
Poultry	Chicken & Noodles	Healthy Choice	260
Meat	Barbecue Steak w Red Potatoes	Healthy Choice	260
Pasta	Tortellini Primavera Parmesan	Healthy Choice	260
Pasta	Sesame Noodles with Vegetables	Smart Ones	260
Pasta	Creamy Rigatoni w Chicken	Smart Ones	260
Pasta	Macaroni & Cheese	Smart Ones	260
Pasta	Butternut Squash Ravioli	Lean Cuisine	260
Other	Santa Fe Rice & Beans	Smart Ones	260
Other	Coconut Chickpea Curry	Lean Cuisine	260
Poultry	Glazed Turkey Tenderloins	Lean Cuisine	270
Poultry	Kung Pao Chicken	Healthy Choice	270
Poultry	Chicken Margherita w Balsamic	Healthy Choice	270
Poultry	Chicken Strips & Sweet Potatoes	Smart Ones	270
Poultry	Thai Style Chicken Rice Noodle	Smart Ones	270
Meat	Salisbury Steak with Mac & Cheese	Lean Cuisine	270
Meat	Sweet & Spicy Harissa Meatballs	Lean Cuisine	270
Meat	Meat Loaf	Smart Ones	270
Pasta	Classic Macaroni & Beef	Lean Cuisine	270
Pasta	Mushroom Mezzaluna Ravioli	Lean Cuisine	270
Other	Vegetable Fried Rice	Smart Ones	280
Other	Asian Pot Stickers	Lean Cuisine	280
Poultry	Sesame Stir Fry with Chicken	Lean Cuisine	280
Poultry	Chicken in Sweet BBQ Sauce	Lean Cuisine	280
Poultry	Apple Cranberry Chicken	Lean Cuisine	280
Poultry	Chicken Fettuccini Alfredo	Healthy Choice	280
Poultry	Grilled Chicken Marinara	Healthy Choice	280
Poultry	Sweet & Spicy Orange Chicken	Healthy Choice	280
Poultry	Chicken Parmesan	Smart Ones	280
Poultry	Turkey Breast with Stuffing	Smart Ones	280

Meat	Beef & Broccoli	Healthy Choice	280
Meat	Meatball Marinara	Healthy Choice	280
Meat	Beef Teriyaki	Healthy Choice	280
Pasta	Spinach Artichoke Ravioli	Lean Cuisine	280
Pasta	Alfredo Pasta w Chicken & Broc	Lean Cuisine	280
Pasta	Three Cheese Ziti Marinara	Smart Ones	280
Pasta	Spinach Artichoke Ravioli	Lean Cuisine	280
Pasta	Alfredo Pasta w Chicken & Broccol	Lean Cuisine	280
Pasta	Linguini with Ricotta & Spinach	Lean Cuisine	280
Pasta	Spaghetti & Meatballs	Healthy Choice	280
Pasta	Spaghetti with Meat Sauce	Smart Ones	280
Other	Vegetable Fried Rice	Smart Ones	280
Other	Asian Pot Stickers	Lean Cuisine	280
Poultry	Chicken with Almonds	Lean Cuisine	290
Poultry	Chicken with Peanut Sauce	Lean Cuisine	290
Poultry	Chicken Fettuccini	Lean Cuisine	290
Poultry	Grilled Chicken Pesto w Veggies	Healthy Choice	290
Poultry	General Tso's Spicy Chicken	Healthy Choice	290
Poultry	Pineapple Chicken	Healthy Choice	290
Poultry	Chicken Enchiladas Suiza	Smart Ones	290
Meat	Swedish Meatballs	Lean Cuisine	290
Seafood	Parmesan Crusted Fish	Lean Cuisine	290
Seafood	Lemon Pepper Fish	Healthy Choice	290
Pasta	Pasta with Swedish Meatballs	Smart Ones	290
Pasta	Pasta with Ricotta & Spinach	Smart Ones	290
Pizza	Thin Crust Cheese Pizza	Smart Ones	290
Other	Cheese & Bean Enchilada	Lean Cuisine	290
Poultry	Sweet & Sour Chicken	Lean Cuisine	300
Poultry	Chicken Fried Rice	Lean Cuisine	300
Poultry	Crustless Chicken Pot Pie	Healthy Choice	300

Poultry	Sweet Sesame Chicken	Healthy Choice	300
Poultry	Chicken Fettuccini	Smart Ones	300
Poultry	Spicy Chicken Strips & Fries	Smart Ones	300
Meat	Classic Meat Loaf	Healthy Choice	300
Seafood	Tortilla Crusted Fish	Lean Cuisine	300
Pasta	Garlic Sesame Noodles with Beef	Lean Cuisine	300
Pasta	Tortellini with Red Pepper Sauce	Lean Cuisine	300
Pasta	Broccoli Cheddar Rotini	Lean Cuisine	300
Pasta	Three Cheese Macaroni	Smart Ones	300
Poultry	Orange Chicken	Lean Cuisine	310
Poultry	Chicken Tikka Masala	Lean Cuisine	310
Poultry	Chicken Strips & Fries	Smart Ones	310
Meat	Spicy Beef & Bean Enchilada	Lean Cuisine	310
Pasta	Lasagna Florentine	Smart Ones	310
Pasta	Traditional Lasagna Meat Sauce	Smart Ones	310
Pasta	Three Cheese Ziti w Meatballs	Smart Ones	310
Pizza	French Bread Pepperoni Pizza	Lean Cuisine	310
Other	Spicy Beef & Bean Enchilada	Lean Cuisine	310
Poultry	Chicken Pecan	Lean Cuisine	320
Poultry	Chicken Fried Rice	Healthy Choice	320
Meat	Sweet & Spicy Korean Beef	Lean Cuisine	320
Pizza	Farmers Market Pizza	Lean Cuisine	320
Pizza	Margherita Pizza	Lean Cuisine	320
Other	Cheese & Fire-Roasted Tamale	Lean Cuisine	330
Poultry	Sesame Chicken	Lean Cuisine	330
Poultry	Mango Chicken w Coconut Rice	Lean Cuisine	330
Poultry	Country Fried Chicken	Healthy Choice	330
Meat	Philly Steak and Cheese Panini	Lean Cuisine	330
Pizza	Supreme Pizza	Lean Cuisine	330
Other	Cheese & Fire-Roasted Tamale	Lean Cuisine	330

Other	Asian Pot Stickers	Healthy Choice	340
Poultry	Chicken Club Panini	Lean Cuisine	350
Poultry	Chicken Spinach Mushroom Panini	Lean Cuisine	350
Poultry	Chicken Parmigiana	Healthy Choice	360
Poultry	Sweet & Sour Chicken	Healthy Choice	390

APPENDIX B
Frozen Food Safety

Increasingly, food giants like ConAgra, Nestlé and others that supply Americans with processed foods concede that they cannot ensure the safety of their food products. Frozen foods pose a particularly serious safety problem because unsuspecting consumers buy frozen foods for their convenience and incorrectly believe that cooking frozen foods is a matter of taste – not safety.

Still the food industry says that extensive outbreaks of food-borne illness are rare, even though it is well-known that most of the millions of cases of food-borne illness every year go unreported or are not traced to the source. For example, each year approximately 40,000 cases of salmonella poisoning are reported in the United States – but perhaps as many as one million cases go unreported. (Salmonella is a type of bacteria most often found in poultry, eggs, unprocessed milk, meat and water.) Recently salmonella pathogens in some frozen meals have sickened thousands of people. How could this happen? First, the supply chain for ingredients in processed foods – from flour to fruits and vegetables to flavorings – is becoming more complex and global in the drive to keep food costs down. As a result, government and industry officials concede that almost every food ingredient is now a potential carrier of pathogens. A further complication is that a large number of food companies subcontract processing work to save money and don't require suppliers to test for pathogens. In fact, companies often don't even know who is supplying their ingredients.

In addition, many frozen-food manufacturers have stopped cooking their products at high temperatures, a tactic they call the "kill step," which is intended to eliminate any lingering microbes. Frequently this process step turns some of the frozen food ingredients into mush. So, instead the "kill step" has been shifted to consumers. For example, ConAgra has added food safety instructions to its frozen meals, including the Healthy Choice brand. A typical "frozen-food safety" instruction offers this guidance: "Internal temperature needs to reach 165°F as measured by a food thermometer in several spots."

Moreover, General Mills, now advises consumers to avoid microwaves altogether and cook their frozen pizzas only in a conventional oven. **<u>Bottom line</u>**: To be safe, always cook frozen foods so that the internal temperature reaches 165°F as measured by a good food thermometer.

APPENDIX C
Soup Selections

The following lists **canned** soup selections. See the important note at the end of list. The soup listed below were available in supermarkets as of 08/25/2020.

Soup	Calories
Progresso Chicken and Wild Rice	80
Progresso Hearty Chicken and Rotini	90
Progresso Garden Vegetable	90
Progresso Minestrone	110
Progresso Chickarina	110
Progresso Italian Wedding	120
Progresso Split Pea	130
Progresso Tuscan-Style White Bean	130
Progresso Lentil	140
Progresso Tomato Basil	150
Progresso Macaroni & Bean	160
Progresso Hearty Penne	160
Progresso Three Cheese Tortellini	170

*** Important:** When the Daily Meal Plan menu specifies soup, have only one serving (8 ounces) unless stated otherwise. To improve the taste of canned soup, add a teaspoon of grated cheese before heating the soup in a microwave oven. After heating, add ½ teaspoon of olive oil. Stir and serve. These additions enhance the taste, and total about 30 Calories which should be added to the soup calories shown in the table above.

100-Day Super Diet-1200 Cal*
100-Day Super Diet-1500 Cal*
100-Day No-Cooking Diet-1200 Cal*
100-Day No-Cooking Diet-1500 Cal*
90-Day Smart Diet-1200 Cal*
90-Day Smart Diet-1500 Cal*
90-Day No-Cooking Diet - 1200 Cal*
90-Day No-Cooking Diet - 1500 Cal*
90-Day Perfect Diet - 1200 Cal*
90-Day Perfect Diet - 1500 Cal*
60-Day Perfect Diet-1200 Cal*
60-Day Perfect Diet-1500 Cal*
50-Day Flex Diet-1200 Cal*
50-Day Flex Diet-1500 Cal*
30-Day Quick Diet - Women*
30-Day Quick Diet for Men*
30-Day No-Cooking Diet*
30-Day Diet for Women - Metric*
30-Day Diet for Men - Metric*
25 Day Easy Diet-1200 Cal*
25 Day Easy Diet-1500 Cal*
25-Day No-Cooking Diet
10-Day Express Diet
10-Day No-Cooking Diet*
7-Day Diet for Women*
7-Day Diet for Men*
7-Day No-Cooking Diets*
90-Day Gluten-Free Diet-1200 Cal*
90-Day Gluten-Free Diet-1500 Cal*
30-Day Gluten-Free Quick Diet*
30-Day Gluten-Free No-Cooking Diet*
7-Day Diet for Women - Metric*
7-Day Diet for Men - Metric
7-Day Gluten-Free Express Diet*
7-Day Gluten-Free No-Cooking Diet*
90-Day Vegetarian Diet-1200 Cal*
90-Day Vegetarian Diet-1500 Cal*
30-Day Vegetarian Diet*
7-Day Vegetarian Diet*
Weight Loss for Women*
Weight Loss for Women - Metric
Weight Loss for Women - UK
Weight Loss for Men*
Maximum Weight Loss - 1200 Cal*
Maximum Weight Loss - 1500 Cal*

Weight Loss for Men - Metric*
Maximum Weight Loss- 1200 Cal*
Maximum Weight Loss- 1500 Cal*
Weight Control - U.S. Edition*
Weight Control - Metric. Edition
Professional Weight Control Women - U.S.
Professional Weight Control Women - Metric
Professional Weight Control Men - U.S.
Professional Weight Control Men - Metric
Weight Maintenance - U.S. Ed*
Weight Maintenance - Metric. Ed*
Weight Maintenance - UK Ed
Weight Loss for Senior Men*
Weight Loss for Senior Women*
Eat Smart - U.S. Edition*
Eat Smart - Metric Edition
30-Day Mediterranean Diet
Exercise Smart - U.S. Edition*
Exercise Smart - Metric Edition
Exercise Smart - UK Edition*
Total Fitness - U.S. Edition
Total Fitness - Metric Edition
Total Fitness - UK Edition
Total Fitness for Women-U.S. Ed*
Total Fitness for Women - Metric
Total Fitness for Women - UK Ed
Total Fitness for Men - U.S. Ed*
Total Fitness for Men- Metric Ed*
Total Fitness for Men - UK Ed
Senior Fitness - U.S. Edition*
Senior Fitness - Metric Edition*
Senior Fitness - UK Edition*
Computer Diet - U.S. Edition*
Computer Diet - Metric Ed*
Reliable Weight Loss - U.S. Ed
101 Weight Loss Tips*
101 Healthy Eating Tips*
101 Lifelong Fitness Tips*
101 Weight Maintenance Tips
101 Weight Loss Recipes
101 GF Weight Loss Recipes
101 Veggie Weight Loss Recipes*
30-Day Mediterranean Diet*
90-Day Mediterranean Diet - 1200 Cal*
90-Day Mediterranean Diet - 1500 Cal*

* These titles are available as both ebooks and paperbacks. Our ebooks are sold by Amazon, Apple, Google, Barnes & Noble and Kobo, but our paperbacks are only sold by Amazon.

Disclaimer

This book offers general meal planning, nutrition and weight control information. It is not a medical manual and the author does not claim to be medically qualified. The material in this book is not intended to be a substitute for medical counseling. Everyone should have a medical checkup before beginning a weight loss program Moreover, the physician conducting the medical exam should be made aware of and should approve the specific weight control program planned. Additionally, while the author and publisher have made every effort to ensure the accuracy of the information in this book, they make no representations or warranties regarding its accuracy or completeness. Further, neither the author nor publisher assume liability for any medical problems that might result from applying the methods in this book, or for any loss of profit, or any other commercial damages, including but not limited to special, incidental, consequential or other damages, and any such liability is hereby expressly disclaimed.

www.ingramcontent.com/pod-product-compliance
Lightning Source LLC
Chambersburg PA
CBHW031132250726
48655CB00002B/639